Slowly, Gradually, Gently

A Recovery Memoir

Gina Luongo

DEDICATION

For those of us stuck between our old life

and the new one waiting

CONTENTS

INTRODUCTION

In the spring of 2013, doctors discovered a rare cancerous tumor growing on my left femoral head, where the thigh bone meets the hip. To save my life, surgeons had to cut through layers of muscle and remove more than a third of my femur and replace it with a prostheses. As a result of the surgery, I permanently lost three muscles groups largely responsible for walking upright, climbing, and rotating side to side. I was told walking long distances would be impossible without the use of a cane, and no longer would I be able to run, do yoga, rollerblade or any other impact activity. As an active person this was and remains devastating news for me.

This book is a collection of reflections I wrote

while on my difficult road to recovery following surgery. Written largely in the moments as I was experiencing them, these reflections today serve as my recollections of how I coped, endured and gradually arrived at this place of acceptance of where I am today.

I have not altered the names or any identifying characteristics of any of the people mentioned in the book because every single one of them deserves my gratitude and recognition.

1 THE RIDE BEGINS

I hate roller coasters . . . always have, always will. But if someone would have told me that I'd have been thrust onto the highest, bumpiest, fastest and most terrifying ride of my life without a choice, a say, not even an inkling, I would have called them crazy. Me . . . on a roller coaster? You mean the ride with gut-dropping dips, sudden turns and daunting, never ending climbs up to an abyss in the sky, you've got the wrong person. I *never* would've voluntarily signed up for such a thing. Nothing terrifies me more than a roller coaster. And that's exactly where I found myself the morning of March 19, 2013 . . . on the loading dock waiting to board the front seat of one of life's scariest rides ever: Cancer Disaster. And who knew that I wasn't just facing my fear that day but I was about to start living it?

May 25, 2014

2 IN THE MOMENT

When the moment you're experiencing is one of the most unrecognizable of your life, what do you do? Is there a guidebook out there that you can turn to, to instruct how to react to the news that you have cancer? Is there an app for that? Do you turn stone cold, staring straight ahead of you, while the world around you fades into the background? Or, how about the classic reactionary response: denial? Such as, this is not happening to me. I'm fine. I'm healthy. These doctors have it all wrong.

I did none of these things when I first received my diagnosis. Well, not really. That feeling of being frozen in my seat, in my mind, in time . . . *that* washed over me like an unexpected, violent wave. That overwhelming sense of how surreal this moment truly is and how it can't be happening to me, I recall clearly, as if it is happening right now. The look of absolute incredulity coming across my face as my doctor grimaced with his. *It's neuroendocrine carcinoma, Gina.* He announced the words but I thought his eyes revealed more. A look, that at that moment, I knew I'd never forget. His eyes were already expressing their condolences, it seemed. *I'm sorry for your loss,* they were saying. I recognized this look immediately because I remember being on the receiving end of it twenty-three years earlier when my mother was diagnosed with cancer. But this time the message, although unspoken, sounded even more terrifying. It was applying to me and to my life. *You're not going to make it,* is what I was hearing.

So what exactly does someone do in that moment? I've no idea. What I do remember doing was reaching for a pen and that little scrap piece of paper I had stuffed in my purse earlier that day. The one with the appointment time, floor and room number of my scheduled visit. Once I pulled the pen out, I remember unscrewing the lid on it with shaking hands. And then with shallow breath, I recall sounding out the syllables in my head of the diagnosis he had given, the first word foreign to my ears and my vocabulary. Neuroendocrine . . . I remember writing it down quickly as neuro-endocrin, leaving out the silent "e". Carcinoma . . . a no-brainer. I knew from my previous experiences into the cancer world with my mother that a carcinoma started with a "t" and ended with "l", as in *t-e-r-m-i-n-a-l.*

And so he talked. The doctor, that is. What he was saying, I couldn't tell you. I was in a state of shock. My insides were shaking and my breathing felt short. I turned and looked over my right shoulder at my husband Carlo, standing a few feet behind me. His jaw was clenched. His face turned pale. His arms were crossed at his chest. But it was the look in his eyes, too, that I also will never forget. In them, I read *disbelief* and *defeat*, all in the same sentence. I heard his voice choking as he tried to ask a few questions. I think I saw his eyes water. We both felt sucker-punched. We just didn't see this coming.

How, you might ask, couldn't you have seen it coming? After all, you were going into this appointment knowing you were about to receive the results from your biopsy. You'd been waiting for these results for almost two months. And that's just the thing, you see. I always had hope. My results will come back as benign, they just have to, I had thought going in that day. This won't be malignant, I had told myself, it just can't be . . . I'm young; I have a family to raise; I don't feel sick . . . were some of the ways I had justified a diagnosis of benign in my mind. The human spirit wants to live. How could I believe this doctor standing in front of me, sullen-faced and serious, and his tragic message of doom? Or was I just imagining the news of my diagnosis in this way, negative and dooming? Maybe he was hopeful that something could be done to save me but I just didn't hear it, couldn't hear it at that moment?

And so, as we left the doctor's office that early evening what I remember thinking while sitting was *I won't be here this time next year.*

I guess that was what I experienced in that most surreal of moments.

May 26, 2014

3 EVERY LITTLE TWITCH

I'm dizzy. No, lightheaded. No, dizzy. I'm seeing double. Oh my gawd . . . my head is spinning. I think I'm going to fall. Grab the counter, the banister, the desk. Anything, before I fall. What's happening to me? Am I going to die? This is it. I'm really going to die.

Welcome to a day in my new life.

Now I feel a twitch in my back. It's just a twitch . . . for now. It's not actually smack dab in the middle of my back. It's off to the side a bit. You know, right above my left kidney. There it goes again. Another twitch. Oh my gawd. My kidney! That's it . . . the cancer has spread to my kidneys. It must have. Why else would I feel this twitch? What's happening to me? Am I going to die? This is it. I'm really going to die.

I no longer trust my body. It has failed me.

Like a partner who cheats, my body has slowly betrayed me over the course of time. It made me feel I was strong and healthy and secure but beneath the surface it was slyly going about its' own agenda, growing a tumor in the most hidden of crevices.

It squeezes my arm and I wait. I can feel it tightening. The blood pressure monitor belt has become my latest accessory. Not exactly an in vogue wardrobe essential but according to my doctors, a necessary tool I need to monitor my blood pressure for the rest of my life. So I strap it on and press a button. And wait. The results appear. The numbers, as expected, are low. I have low blood pressure. Always have and likely always will. I jot down the reading in my little notebook and repeat the test again. Let's see if those wee numbers will climb a bit. Wait. Keep waiting. Yes . . . a little higher. Third time's a charm, they say. So, let's give it a go. Success! Numbers have risen. Minimally. But at least they haven't decreased. I repeat this ritual on a weekly basis for months. When I review the hastily kept records of my blood pressure readings each week, I begin to see a pattern emerge. I have low blood pressure. Consistently. What does that mean for me? Is this a sign that something is wrong? What's happening to me? Am I going to die? This is it. The writing seems to be on the wall and in my notebook. I'm really going to die.

This cycle of catastrophic thinking is pervasive. Once the trigger is set off by a twitch or a sensation in my body, my mind starts rolling with it. And the more it's allowed to indulge in these unreasonable thoughts, the more convincing they appear to me. *Yes, Gina . . . the cancer is coming back . . . of course it is.* My therapist would say that this hyper vigilance towards my health is an after effect of the trauma I've experienced. I think of those soldiers who return from war and can't stop seeing danger around them, even in the safety of their own homes and surrounded by loved ones. They suffer from it in their own way too.

Sometimes I believe these extreme reactions I'm having are a result of the trust I've lost in this body of mine. Because prior to my diagnosis and throughout all my adult life, I had considered myself strong and fit, healthy and energetic. I'd never smoked and rarely did I drink alcohol. And that little nudge I had begun feeling deep in my left hip two months before seeing a chiropractor about it, I had dismissed as a runner's injury that would go away. Never in a million years would my mind had even gone to a place where cancer was a possibility. I was beyond blind-sided by this diagnosis. And all trust in this warrior body of mine that had previously been there had flown out the window.

Both my body and my mind have wreaked the havoc this disease brings with it. I'm a sufferer of a different kind of war. I imagine many survivors are.

I have another twitch. More like an ache. It's in my lower back area this time. It's a dull ache but the longer I sit here writing this piece the more that it's turning into full out back pain. I stretch in between typing sentences to see if that will ease the pain. I stand up and take a short walk but even that doesn't help. I'll have to ask Sabrina, my physiotherapist, about this latest symptom. Maybe she'll tell me the back pain is related to my tight hip joints. The back is bearing the brunt of the load that your hips would normally. This makes complete sense but my thoughts quickly lure me like bait, away from logic and back to the darkness. I sit here and recall the discouragement of those early days when the original symptoms in my left hip started to manifest; the nudge in the groin, the limp to my step that never went away. Is this low back pain the early signs of a tumor on my right hip this time?

Even as I reread this paragraph I can see how irrational my thoughts get. These symptoms I feel are not even similar to what I was feeling prior to my diagnosis and yet I self-diagnose my symptoms with same conclusion every time: life-threatening. And here I go again: is this a sign that something is wrong? What's happening to me? Am I going to die? Is this it?

Sometimes it feels like I'll never be at peace.

SLOWLY, GRADUALLY, GENTLY

June 2, 2014

.

4 WEEPINESS

I've never understood the word *weepy*. To cry, yes. To wail, definitely. But weepiness? I can't say I remember ever having had bouts of sadness with uncontrollable crying like these, before cancer. I had had episodes of depression where I had cried to relieve the sorrow within: missing my mother, the early days of motherhood marked by sleeplessness and loss of independence, feeling sad over another's tragedy. But those days didn't go on forever. These days, though, seem to.

Among the many lessons cancer has given me includes what emotional pain feels like. What I've learned and am learning is that the pain I feel brought on by the emotions I'm experiencing are as deep and real as the throbbing in my leg muscles at the end of the day. My chest and my heart can only withstand so much heaviness before they seek release. It feels, throughout this past year, that my quivering chin seems to be losing its ability to stop impending tears from flooding my eyes. I am bareback on a horse and have lost hold of the reins. The beast, this disease and the emotional pain it causes, has taken over me.

I cry and I cry. Everyday. Sometimes two or three times a day. Anything or everything can set me off. At times, it's my leg and its' limitations. How I miss bending at the knees to pick up something that I've dropped. What I'd do to jump and jog and climb the stairs again without looking like a baby learning how to climb with the help of an adult behind her. Good leg up first. Stop. Bad leg up next. Stop again. Repeat. I watch my kids tumbling and bouncing on the backyard trampoline and cry while watching them. I'll never be able to join them in there. I'm a woman who feels her body is aging well before it should. In public, I take note of all the cane walkers out there and so far, I'm the youngest I see. I cry. Doing any sort of modified physical activity such as spinning class or walking around the neighborhood with my urban walking poles will more often than not trigger the weepiness. The thoughts in my head, like *look at you . . . look at how disabled you've become . . . how did this happen . . .* will do it.

I put sunglasses on, even on an overcast day, to hide the tears. And those sunglasses also protect me from the looks of pity I get from others watching me. People who knew the old Gina, the one who never used to stop running and moving, is disabled now. Those stares or kind offers to lend a hand to the disabled Gina, those cause me to weep. *How did this happen to me?* I want to scream.

Other times, it's thoughts of my past life that plague me; the loss of my independence, my once-strong physical capabilities, the further slaughtering of my innocent and hopeful notions about life. What about the loss of that ignorance-is-bliss state of being? I had no way of knowing what was lurking ahead for me. How did this all turn so fast on me? One day I was living a typical existence like everyone else and the next day it was taken from me. I cry for those lost days.

Can I ever make peace with my new reality? Do I have it in me to accept this broken Gina as the new Gina and love her just the same? Or maybe more? Will my chin one day quiver less in the presence of these sad thoughts? Will the pity ever go away? I've no idea but for now I understand what it feels like. Weepiness. I feel it all the time.

June 3, 2014

5 THE LIMP

First off, it's not painful. Second, I like to think of it as more of a wobble than a limp. A limp is how I walked one time years ago when I banged my knee up bad enough that I couldn't bend it. Or, once when I cut the bottom of my foot on something sharp and shouldn't have been walking on it. That time, I limped. And as I did, I recall my face contorting in a weird way, conveying the discomfort I was feeling down at the other end of my body. Each step was an effort: unnatural and painful.

Today I wobble. When my cane is cast aside or too far out of reach, I move across the room part like a penguin and part like a baby taking its first steps. I use my arms to center me before I move. And then those arms swing low on each side of my hips to maintain my balance. Each time I step with my left foot, my body dips to the left as if it's a teeter-totter dropping on its end. Then, when my right foot takes its step, the seesaw balances itself out . . . but not for long. That darned left foot has to do its thing all over again. So I wobble along painlessly.

But not hesitantly. I understand that my wobble makes me look less able, more disabled. I realize that I walk a lot slower than I used to and that it tires me out twice as fast. I'm self-aware enough to know that I'm being watched. That people look at me and wonder why I'm walking with a cane. Sometimes I dread getting up from a seated position to grab something quickly, like a fork from the cutlery drawer. All that work for what should be a quick second's work. Those middle of the night bathroom trips? The bane of my existence (and of my husband's too, I'm sure).

A wobble does not go quietly into the good night. My left foot shuffles along the floor while my right foot, bearing most of my body weight, hits the hardwood floor heavily and loudly. Who can fall back asleep after that?

But *you're walking*, you're probably thinking. *You could have lost your whole leg or entire hip*, you might even say. And I'd agree with you in a heartbeat. I *am* walking on the pool deck to get inside the pool. I *am* walking into Chapters with my daughters by my side. I *am* walking to the stove and around my kitchen to make my family our meals. I am walking my way around my new life that on some days resembles my old life but not entirely. Because now I wobble along much shorter distances. I'm here.

June 13, 2014

6 DATES

Why can't I get over the dates? In the grand scheme, aren't they just arbitrary days and numbers we attach to events? Wedding anniversaries, birthdays, the death of loved ones. Some of us don't even need a reminder that an important event is coming up because we just know.

Why is it, though, that I remember every single significant date in my cancer ordeal? Come to think of it, I can even recall what I was wearing on those dates, who was in the room with me and even what the weather outside was like. These details are etched on my mind, tattooed there. Oh, how I wish they weren't.

March 19th, April 15th, April 22nd, April 29th,

May 14th, May 29th, June 10th, June 20th, October 9th, January 20th, March 3rd. I see now but couldn't see then that these days, like stepping-stones, were guiding me along a never-before travelled pathway. With each date that passed and each step I took, I was heading somewhere. An end? A beginning? I hadn't a clue. But how I remember the blows that hit me, that blindsided me, in fact, each and every time. On all of these days, I was unprepared for what was waiting for me. Sometimes, it was news I wasn't expecting to hear or diagnoses I didn't fully understand. One particular day, I recall with relief and lots of gratitude, handed me what felt like a winning lottery ticket; a hopeful and optimistic action plan (Thank you, Dr. Monika). The thing is there were many other days on this journey but why can't I erase these particular ones from my memory?

Maybe it's because these dates remind me of a time in my life when these days in particular had been nothing special or out of the ordinary.

These were days in my life like all the others: went to work, then home, to sleep and woke up again. Normalcy. Some semblance of control, however illusory that control was, I now see. These were days that were unmarked by symptoms or disease. They were dates that weren't indicated on my calendar as appointments with an oncologist or a therapist of some kind. They are dates that in my before-cancer life remind me of the bliss of not knowing of what was lying ahead for me. I guess the old cliché is right. You can't go back.

I think of the families of the victims of tragic world events like 9/11 or the disappearance of the Malaysian flight and understand how the pages of the calendar now mar their lives. One morning they woke up beside their loved ones and by nightfall they were abandoned by them. Every day lived without them counts as one day closer to the wretched anniversary of their senseless deaths. I know I'm not the only one who hates anniversaries. I just wish, as these families do, that none of it would've happened in the first place.

So here I am on the eve of my first post-surgery anniversary, writing this reflection and thinking about how each of these dates were leading me somewhere. And it's here. June 18th, 2014. I'm here today, knowing what I know, feeling the way I'm feeling and understanding so much more about life and pain and struggle and joy and surrender than I did on June 18th, 2013 and on June 18th, 2012 and even on June 18th, 2011. Maybe the pain of remembering these dates will begin to fade with time. Or not.

June 18, 2014

7 FIRST RESPONDERS

Shortly after the 2012 Newton school shootings, I was watching a news story on one of the American channels about the aftermath of the shocking tragedy when I heard a phrase that stuck with me. It went something like "when catastrophe hits, focus on the helpers."

The news segment was reporting on a Newtown resident whose home was steps away from the elementary school where the killings took place. Immediately following the shooting spree, this man took in and protected five or six young children who had fled the school and needed refuge until their parents were notified. Stories of the helpers after 9/11 and the helpers after Hurricane Katrina and the behind-the-scenes helpers of many horrific tragedies followed. Focus on the helpers. They're the ones who pull us through.

Here's the story about my helpers. I believe they helped pulled me through the tsunami wave that blindsided me. I was blessed to have an army of willing hands and loving hearts who came through for my family and me during our time of crisis. And what is most amazing about these people is that they all somehow knew, instinctively or not, how to be with me, a person drowning in the middle of a tsunami. They were there on the shores when the wave hit, holding branches out for me to grasp and clearing the debris from my path, protecting me from further harm. They remained silent in the midst of all the noise around me. They focused on my needs, both physical and emotional, and delivered in spades. And what's even more incredible is that not one of them ever showed me how worried and scared they were about me when they were with me. I felt only their presence and their love and their genuine desire to want to help me. How lucky was I . . . and still am.

My inner circle consisted of my two sisters, Rina and Daniela, my godmother Emma, my cousin Rina D and my dear friends Pina and Liliana. Any of the six, or sometimes all of them, got the first call or text once we left a doctor's appointment. That's how they became my inner circle. I knew I wanted them to be the first to know whatever news I had to share. During those first few weeks, taking hospital shifts, shaving my legs, driving me places, making meals for me and my family, helping me with my bedpan (!), sitting with me over tea and allowing me to nap were ways they truly helped me when I needed it. A phone call or a simple text saying *thinking of you* worked too. They were my first responders.

Thank you to each of them for their strength when my own was waning. Thank you, thank you, and thank you. I love you all.

June 23, 2014

8 ANNABEL'S GRADUATION DAY

I feel so much honor and love in my heart right now that I could just burst. This is what true gratitude feels like. I'm so thankful to have Annabel Vicky Ricci as my daughter. And her little sister Karina is the apple of my eye. What a gift these two are to me.

An hour ago, at Annabel's grade 5 graduation ceremony, she was standing up in front of an audience of many to collect the Principal's Award. And the words the Principal chose to describe why Annabel was the recipient of this award touched all of us sitting in the audience. And as a parent listening to accolades and adjectives describing my daughter, I was beaming with pride. Not because I'm her mother but because every word said rang true. Annabel is a very special person. She is as kind as she is gentle. She is responsible and trustworthy. She roots for the underdog. All the values her father and I hold as important have become Annabel's values, too. What parent wouldn't be proud of a child like this?

Then there's Karina who, when I look at and listen to her, I see and hear visions of my younger self. She reminds me of myself as a child. Some days it feels like I've been cloned, but for the better. Karina is stronger, wiser and wittier, than I ever was.

Today's graduation was among the best moments in my life. I'm so grateful and peaceful for everything I have today. Exactly a year ago I was lying in an Intensive Care unit in the worst shape of my life.

Time has been healing.

June 24, 2014

SLOWLY, GRADUALLY, GENTLY

9 THE PAIN IN MY LEG

I want to try to describe the pain I'm feeling in my left leg right now. To start, it doesn't feel anything like my right leg: pain-free, light, irrelevant.

From the top of my left thigh to the tip of my kneecap, the muscles in my leg are throbbing. They squeeze and then release. They pound for a while and then relent. To the touch, they are sore. Taut like pulled elastic. With my hand, I reach down and rub my thigh up and down hoping to loosen the tension. Then I take my hands and place them on either side of my thigh and shake. Shake the flesh of my thigh and feel the muscle loosen. I do anything I can for that release of pain.

I stand up and immediately feel that dreaded pinch right where my thigh meets my pelvis. It's an excruciating, burning pinch that sometimes is strong enough to cause me to shriek. My face wears the pain, as does my leg. I push my thumb deep into the area hoping to control the pinch which rarely works. So I carry myself to the couch, lift my battered leg onto the cushion of the sofa and breathe out. I surrender.

My leg wins. Respite and stillness it gets. Just when I think I can carry on activities as an able-bodied person, like unloading the dishwasher or going for a walk around the block, my leg tells me otherwise. *Not today,* it says. Three steps forward, two back, it seems, reminding me of a child standing at a buffet whose eyes are bigger than his stomach's . . . I'm left wanting so much more than this body can handle. I have big eyes for all things mobility-related. I yearn to hike in a forest or stroll through an unexplored neighborhood. I crave a long walk like some crave a tall drink. I watch people on paddleboards and imagine myself on top of one wading through calm waters. What I'd do to feel the breeze through my hair while jogging on a cool, autumn morning again. Like a blunt force, pain and restriction of movement block these desires but still leave me wanting.

Last night, when the pain got really bad, I took a Tylenol. It's not something I often do. But last night I found it necessary to take, especially before those wretched middle-of-the-night thoughts would have taken over. I sought refuge in a pill that would relax me and dull the throbbing in my leg before my mind and sad thoughts threatened to keep me awake longer. Today I will turn to another pain management strategy I've adopted: meditation. I'll lie on my couch and breathe deeply, watching through my mind's eye, the pain in my body. I will locate the pain and breathe my way in and then out of it. I will not try to control the aching but will watch it instead. If the pain moves from my thigh to my shin, I'll follow it with both breath and attention. I won't wish it away. I'll accept its presence here in my body and breathe my way through it.

I know of no other way to live with this pain. I don't have my physiotherapist or massage therapist with me at all times to turn to for pain relief. Arnica gel and A535 cream I use when the pain becomes intolerable. Carlo helps by giving me deep rubs along my thigh whenever I ask. I embrace the pain-free days that come to me and bear down on the pain-laden ones and I try to remember to thank the universe for both. As much as the pain depresses me, I know that it also humbles me by reminding me of how to live: one day at a time.

Living with pain was never in my life's plan (I doubt it would be in anybody's). But sometimes learning to accept this new life of mine hurts more than the pain.

July 7, 2014

10 IT TAKES A VILLAGE

It all started with Carm, my chiropractor and cousin. He passed the baton onto Dr. Jay Wunder, the orthopedic oncologist, who ran with it for a while and then conceded to the expertise of a different type of specialist, Dr. Monika Kryzynowska, a medical oncologist specializing in neuroendocrine tumors. She sprinkled the wand with her own brand of magic dust and then shared it with Dr. Ezzat, an oncological endocrinologist. Not long after, the geneticist Dr. Morel joined in too. I was running the circuit for a while being referred from chiropractor to orthopod to oncologist to endocrinologist. I figured that collectively, these doctors probably shared a mountain of experience in assessing and treating conditions and disease. I felt like I was in great, capable hands and still do.

Speaking of hands . . . enter Sabrina Chow, my physiotherapist. It's in hers where my battered leg and wavering spirit have found themselves every week for the past year. While she's been working on helping me to improve my range of movement and rebuild leg strength, she has inadvertently been treating my beaten-up psyche at the same time. Sabrina has been witness to this slow recovery of mine in all its stages but most importantly, she has seen the psychological damage this experience has done to me. I have probably shed more tears lying on Sabrina's table than anywhere else. I've been a tough case on her workload. But her empathy and patience seem to be working. I am better than I was that day when I met her a year ago hobbling in on two crutches with a smile nowhere in sight.

There have been a few other angels in the health care world who've joined me at some point along this journey. Like my family doctor, Karyn Sheldon, entering the battlefield after the battle was fought. It was she who was there to help me pick up the pieces and to make sense of the remnants I was left with. With her careful words, she helped me apply for long-term disability benefits so that I could have the time off work that I needed to heal. Then there was my massage therapist Laura Brossman and her exceptional hands that I now wish could've arrived on the scene earlier. Writhing in pain from the tightness in my legs and back, Laura's hands have provided relief and refuge. This is a woman who literally has a very special touch, much like my other therapists.

Whether you're in the eye of the storm or clinging on a raft as the waters begin to calm, I've learned that different situations call for different kinds of help. While my doctors and surgeons were there when the storm hit, in the months afterward I was left floating in an ocean of grief, drowning in tears. In the darkness of the waters, I couldn't see the horizon. Approaching the first anniversary of my diagnosis and the dates of my surgeries, I was experiencing what I now understand to be post-traumatic stress symptoms. Extreme hyper vigilance around all areas of my health, horrible nightmares, gripping anxiety, pervasive and depressing thoughts and the relentless replaying in my mind of the events leading up to my diagnosis from a year ago as if on a continuous loop or feed like you'd see on news channel. I knew that I needed a different kind of help. Something that was less medical and more therapeutic. My leg may have been a mess but I think that at that time my spirit was more in ruins.

And that's when Janice Carere, my therapist, came on board and took a seat next to me on my raft. Taking one end of my oar, Janice helped me wade through the waters of my sorrow. Together we revisited the site of my trauma and unearthed an ironic discovery. Back in 1990, three days before my mother died, she had gotten out of her hospital bed, had fallen and broken her left femoral head. The tumor that was found in my own body twenty-three years later was on my left femoral head. So you see, much work was to be done around embodied grief. And loss. And anxiety. Let's not forget anger. But above all else, it was the sadness I couldn't shake. So Janice and I discussed all of these and she helped me put my traumatic experience with cancer in a context that I could live with. She showed me how different my story is than my mother's was. She helped me understand how the fall, as I called it, from my previously uber-controlled life of career, family, fitness, intellectual and creative pursuits was really an awakening about how to live. We don't have control over our lives as much as we think we do. To truly live, openly and fully, we must surrender. My new mantra, however cliché, has become *one day at a time.*

I can't end this reflection on the health care professionals who treated and continue to care for me without a mention of Margaret Bangia, my spinning class instructor. I remember the first morning I showed up to her class, forearm crutch in position, and her asking me about what had happened to me. She immediately called me an inspiration, something that I never saw myself ever being referred to. And every single class after that one, Margaret would introduce me to the class as such. Me? An inspiration? I'd never looked at myself that way. Margaret's patience and encouragement helped propel me forward in my recovery by allowing myself to see that I could join the outside world again in a fitness class, however modified it needed to be for me.

All of these people were lifelines to me. I hope they realize how much they helped me get through very difficult days. They all made a difference.

July 10, 2014

11 MOM'S STORY

I've realized that this collection of reflections I've been writing about wouldn't be and couldn't be understood without sharing the context of my story within my mother's. But as I share her story with you I realize I'm telling it through the eyes of the eighteen year old that I was when she died but with the voice and perspective of the forty-two year old I am today.

In my mind's eye I see Mom wobbling along on her one good leg (very much like I limp around these days) as if she is right in front of me. Time and years that have passed don't come into play, she is here right in front of me. I smell the sweet scent of my mother and I feel the softness of the skin around her neck like I used to do when we'd nuzzle up with each other lying on the couch. If I stop everything that I'm doing right now and sit still for a while, I can feel her here beside me, in this room, and I feel comforted and safe. I become eighteen years old all over again.

Forty-two year old me, though, has a story to share. In some ways, it's a medical one. But it's also a story about the power of genetics, and the glue that binds me with my family.

In the summer of 1989, my forty-two year old mother, Vicky, began to complain of a bad backache. Right away you can see the similarities in our ages. The pain she was experiencing at first was somewhat tolerable. Visits to a chiropractor for a few weeks were not helping to ease the increasingly more sleepless nights she was beginning to have. I remember her picking me up one August night from my part-time job at TD Bank and she was clutching the steering wheel close to her chest because leaning back and putting pressure on her back was painful. Fast-forward to early September and her family doctor sent her for an x-ray, which revealed a massive tumor lodged on the upper left side of her back.

The date was September 14, 1989. A day none of us will ever forget. My sisters and I all came home from school to find her crying. She told us she had a cancerous tumor. Like typical teenagers, my sister Rina and I retreated immediately to our bedrooms. I think we were reeling from the shock of the news. Even as I type this last sentence I recognize what a selfish response that was. Neither of us comforted her or hugged her or just stayed with her. She must have been so terrified and we did nothing to ease her fear. One of my life's regrets.

In October she underwent major surgery to remove the tumor. We were told she had had a rare cancer of the adrenal gland (so rare that it typically afflicts 1 in 500,000 people). Doctors were able to remove seventy percent of the tumor and were hoping follow up radiation and chemotherapy would help shrink the rest. It's funny how we always remember the stats, the numbers, and the dates. It's like they're stamped in ink on our minds. But by January of 1990, she began to complain of pain in her legs and in her back once again. Bad pain. Ferocious pain. Further tests revealed the cancer had spread to her bones. After she died later that year, my dad had told us that it was in January when the doctors had told my mother to get her affairs in order. The diagnosis had been terminal. But as teenagers, my sisters and I hadn't been told any of this. In the following months, as her health was failing, we were learning to take on more responsibility. We were losing our mother but didn't know it because Mommy dying seemed the most unfathomable possibility to us. How were we to have known that her body was slowly dying when she continued to fight her battle like a champion? Enduring bouts of sickening chemo, radiation, trips to faith healers, pilgrimages to saints, surgeries, Mommy tried anything and everything to save her life. Or, knowing what she knew at the time, she was fighting to prolong her precious life as long as possible. She fought hard not to leave us motherless but the battle was just bigger than her. At the age of forty-three, she died on November 14, 1990, fourteen months after her initial diagnosis.

Twenty-three years later Dr. Ezzat, an endocrinologist at Princess Margaret Hospital who I as referred to but I wasn't sure why at the time, was the person who dropped the bomb on me. Without genetic testing to confirm it nor not having looked at my mother's medical reports, he couldn't say for sure but he had some suspicions that my cancer was genetically linked to my mother's. Bombshell. And knowing this, I knew I'd never be the same again. Because even if his suspicions turned out to be incorrect, the truth is that we would never know for sure. Mom was gone. And I'm left wondering. That roller coaster I was on had hit one of its peaks that afternoon. Scared as hell, I was holding on for dear life.

July 15, 2014

12 THE CANE

It drops again. As it falls, it makes its familiar sound upon hitting the ground. A clunk, loud and clear. I've heard the sound so often that I can hear it falling even when it's not. And if you're not used to it or ready for it, the sound can startle you. But it's a new part of my life, among other things. I'm getting used to it. It's coming up to six months since I've been using my cane. Before that, I was on a forearm crutch and before that, I was using one crutch. And before that, I was using two crutches. And even before that, I was using a walker to get around. So, I try to think of the cane as a gradual upgrade in status. It feels like I've gradually been weaning myself from the various walking aids that I've been dependent on for over a year. The cane seems the lightest dosage I've been on.

The cane has become more than just a walking stick. For me, it's a symbol as well, of a battle fought. Most forty-two-year-olds you see walking around are not using a cane. When people in public see me they must wonder what happened. Did she have knee surgery? Was it a car accident? A bad fall? What ordeal has she been through? Some ask. But the majority don't. And, depending on my mood or the circumstances of where I am or even who's asking, I share one of a few versions of my story. To some, I reply very quickly with "oh, I've had surgery" and wave goodbye. To others, I might say that I'm still recovering from surgery and need the cane for a while longer. A slightly more detailed response, but not really. If the person probes and asks what type of surgery, then I gauge how much I feel like sharing at that time. If my children are with me when I'm asked, I never give any more information other than it was hip surgery. Why do they need to hear the story again? If I'm alone, I may give a brief synopsis: rare tumor found on top of femur, had to be removed so part of my femur was cut off and replaced with a prostheses, learning to walk again. Period. Then I take note of the look on the person's face. A combination of shock mixed with pity. I'm used to it by now. Time to move on and so I hobble away as quickly as I can. If I stay long enough, I might hear some compassionate words like "you've been through a lot" or "you look great."

If the cane is an indication of adversity, for me it has also become a sign of disability. With the cane, I can walk easily and justifiably into a public washroom with the handicapped symbol posted on it. I can use the shower stall at the pool equipped with the bars without getting any odd stares from onlookers. I can now park close to the front at the mall, theatre, library, doctor's office, and restaurants with my disabled parking pass. Someone asked me if people stare me down as I'm pulling into one of those blue parking spaces because I look so young to be using one of those parking areas. And I do get curious looks until I open my door and wave my cane in the air, making me a legitimate user of the space. But if this sounds like I'm celebrating the comforts of public accessibility, I'm not. In fact, I hate it. How I wish I wasn't disabled. I'd love to take the stairs again if I could. I'm too young to live with restrictions and limitations. I'm working my body hard to get to the day when I no longer need to take the elevator one floor up.

Walking with a cane means I always have to plan ahead. A certain amount of spontaneity is lost when you have to plan how you will walk down the stairs into the pool area carrying a towel, a water bottle, goggles and cap and any swimming gear like a flutter board using only one hand. The cane permanently takes up the use of one hand so going for a walk with a coffee in hand is never an easy feat. If my daughter reaches to hold my free hand when we're out in public, I quickly have to pass any bags I'm carrying to someone else to carry. This past year, I wasn't able to carry a birthday cake with lit candles on it to my birthday girls or take over a tray of any kind anywhere. I can no longer carry laundry baskets, big boxes or grocery bags from the car. A lot of my old life rituals are lost. Some tell me that they're not lost but have just gone away for a while. I'm not sure. Sometimes it feels like this cane has joined my body as a third leg, or an outfit accessory, stuck to me like a tattoo. I have to learn to make peace with the fact that it'll likely be permanent.

If there is any positive spin I can take on this whole cane business it's this: this cane has reminded me a few important life lessons that my life had been trying to tell me all along (but I wasn't listening). *Slow down. Pause. Take one step at a time.* No longer can I pummel through my days rushing from one place to the next like I used to. I can't skip stairs to get to the top more quickly anymore. The stair banister and the cane remind me I can only take one step at a time.

I recall the old cliché about life not being a race but a marathon. One day I'll get there, I hope. With my cane, I guess.

September 10, 2014

13 TERRY FOX DAY

It started with a pledge. A promise I had made to my sister and to myself. But really, I think it began with a vision I had had in my mind exactly one year ago to the day. I saw myself walking among others in the 2014 Terry Fox Run. I had actually imagined myself up on my feet and moving on my own. What a fool. At the time I made the promise I used to be seated for eighty percent of my day: on the couch, in my wheelchair, in the passenger seat of the car. The idea of giving myself a far off goal like walking again in a charity walk seemed inspirational. And even though I've wholeheartedly adopted the "one day at a time" mantra since this all happened to me, I was hoping that the future would have brought some type of miraculous turnaround and I actually would've been walking along the trails of Boyd Park yesterday among the other participants. I was sitting in my wheelchair instead.

Why did I even go on the charity walk, I ask myself. Perhaps I wouldn't be feeling like I am right now if I'd have skipped it instead. On some level, I knew it was going to be a difficult day watching the runners around me run. Watching them all jog by me, I studied the ways their hips lifted them up while their legs carried them forward. I was in awe of the moving human body. I stared at the sweat rolling down their faces and envied it. It's been so long since I've been able to work up that intense a sweat. I remembered that high I used to get when jogging and knew that those runners were experiencing it yesterday. My chin started to quiver and my eyes welled with tears. So, I turned my attention over to the walkers and began admiring the tone of their calf muscles and rhythm of their swinging arms. The fact that they were all walking upright and without the aid of something left me wanting to do the same so badly.

Sitting in a wheelchair allows me time to observe the world around me from a different perspective. I can study people's walk or outline their body shape. I revel in watching the human body do the things it does like bend, stretch, tiptoe, flex, move. Sitting in the chair, I feel closer to nature. I look at the ground a lot more and then I look up and observe the ways the trees sway in the wind. I notice that my senses come more alive when my body sits still. But sitting in the chair also gives me more time alone with my thoughts. And then sadness seeps into my heart, a slow descent, like it did yesterday, as I watched the runners run. I know I'll never be able to run again.

Why am I having such a hard time accepting my new reality? Fifteen months after the fact and

I'm still mourning the loss of speed and freedom of movement I used to love about running. Will the pain of loss ease as more time passes? I tell myself to find some other activity that I can do and then do it a lot. Maybe a love affair with it will ensue? Then I think about all the people who have to give up doing what they love for various reasons. I know I'm not alone. I just wish I had a few more years with it, I guess. I'm sure Terry Fox wished for even more.

So, I've decided I'm not going to pledge to do anything or join or participate in any event so far in advance again. I cannot afford the luxury of imagining myself as I was before or better than before. I can only focus on what I have today and what I'm able to do right now. I realize my mourning process is far from over so I'll mourn. I'm going to continue to cry when I feel like it because my tears somehow comfort me and get me through the moment. And whenever I watch a runner on the sidewalk, I'll try to pretend I'm in their shoes for just a few moments so I can feel the breeze through my hair and the fresh air in my lungs.

If you're reading this and you're a runner, jog a little lap for me and thank the universe that your body is working today.

September 15, 2014

14 TIME TO HEAL

I've been off work since April 18, 2013. Today is September 18, 2014. I'm on an extended medical leave and continue to be paid by my employer's Long Term Disability coverage. I realize how fortunate I am to have written that last sentence. I've repeatedly said that my cancer ordeal has brought small blessings wrapped up in interesting ways. An extended time off to recuperate and heal from major surgery without the stress of financial worries brought on by loss of income is definitely one of these gifts.

Maybe because I've been off work for this long a period of time, people who haven't seen me in a while have begun asking me if I'm back at work yet. A valid question and one I know that

I've asked people I know who were off work for a while following an illness or accident. When I tell people that I'm still off work, most of them say they're happy to hear because "no one needs the added stress that work inevitably brings." Or, they'll say something like "take all the time you need to get stronger" or "stay off work as long as you can". And I know they're right. I'm fairly certain that adding work stress onto my recovery process wouldn't be easy at this point.

Everyday I work on walking upright and trying to squeeze these damned glutes, among other exercises. Managing to get from points A to B while carrying a bag or something in my hand is a major preparation exercise. How can I carry a water bottle while using my cane and hold my daughter's hand at the same time? Am I going to get my left sock on today in two tries or ten? Getting in and out of my car now takes much longer than it ever used to. The automatic movements that people take for granted everyday

I no longer can. Getting up a flight of stairs is now a half day's worth of energy expended. Picking up something that has fallen on the floor is more work than you realize. But I try not to complain because moving is so much better than not moving. It's just that since moving successfully is still a work in process for me, adding career responsibilities on top of all this right now would probably not be in my best interest.

Or would it?

People who enjoy their work often say that work gives them purpose. These same people sometimes say that going to work stimulates them. That having a routine is important for them. That work provides them with identity. Work offers distraction from the stresses of their personal lives. Of course, work also provides income.

I wonder if, just maybe, going back to work would help my healing? Work would distract me from all the thinking that I do and would steer my focus away from every twinge or ache my body experiences setting me off in panic mode.

I've been finding myself thinking more and more about the distance that has grown between my current life of recovery and healing and my work life. A year and a half is a long time to not be within my "working mind" and this disconnect sometimes overwhelms me with sadness. I miss interacting with colleagues. I miss using my mind to solve problems and organize thoughts around work. I miss getting in my car every morning and having a place I need to be. My physiotherapist says this is a positive sign. If I'm thinking about work, then I must be getting better, she says. She recalls the first few months of working with me and me never even mentioning that I had a career. Maybe all this time off is helping to heal my internal and external wounds.

But then fear sets in. The position I left might still be waiting for me but I'm no longer the same person I was when I left that position seventeen months ago. I've lost some stamina, of course. My energy levels are certainly not the same as they used to be. I honestly don't think I could keep up the pace required of the position. How could I possibly fit in my new regimen of frequent hospital tests and screening followed by specialists' appointments with that position? I'd alone use up my allotted sick days within the first few months of returning to work. The stress I'd undertake in the transition back to work would set me back.

So, in the mean time, I guess I could just allow myself to miss work. And wonder about work. And try visualizing my new self back in some type of work. This means healing is happening. But if I stop and listen to myself for just a second what I'm hearing is that I'm really not ready to return yet. I need to continue to nurture myself with calm and quiet days doing things that I want to do. At this moment in time, I think this is what my body and my life need: more self-love.

September 18, 2014

15 FAITH

I want to build a new life. I want to start fresh on a clean slate. I want to see what my life can become. But I feel so lost. I don't know where to begin building this new life.

I ask myself if this idea I have in my mind of a new life, a new beginning, is just a fantasy that I've created in my mind over the past year and a half? How I wish that this vision that I have of my less-than-perfect, rehabilitated leg carrying me forward into a new day, one filled with exciting beginnings, were here. I remind myself everyday of the courage I need to believe that the best is yet to come. I tell myself that even though things don't feel like they're moving forward, they actually are. They have to be. Nothing stays the same. More importantly, I repeat the words "Trust the universe, not yourself" when I'm feeling lost, like today. "Stop trying to take control. Allow the universe to do what it needs to do", the woman in my guided meditation practice says. She's right. But I'm not listening well.

Where was I a year ago? I look back at my journal to find out. The entry from October 1, 2013 was about one of my doctor visits. *"Dr. Wunder impressed with the two or three steps I took today,"* the notes say. This morning, I walked, limp fully intact, in and out of my health club without my cane and I swam thirty laps while I was there. More than two or three steps from this day last year. Progress. Lucky for me, things *have* moved forward and I'm grateful.

Then I flip ahead a bit to the October 7th 2013 journal entry where I wrote: *"Crying again in physio today. I was attempting to do a full leg lift, (so MIGHTY hard) I couldn't lift my leg up at all. Damian (physio assistant) had to help me lift my leg for a ten-minute exercise. I'm reminded how far I've fallen. I'm disabled now.*" Ironically, I was in physio just two days ago working on this exact same exercise . . . and I still couldn't lift my leg. Same physio bed, a year later, and still feeling disabled. So, maybe some things don't move along as much as I hope.

I spend a few minutes skimming more journal entries. I'm reading the stories and seeing a roller coaster ride of emotions filled with ups and downs. There've been days when I've been on a high, hopeful and positive about a great new life ahead of me, ripe with possibility and opportunity. Then, there are days, like today, where I see the fog lurking in my thoughts. My life feels stripped down to physio appointments, countless leg stretches, managing pain and learning to walk again. Anxious to return to the land of the well but not able to get there quite yet, I feel like I'm not moving forward. And if I'm not moving forward, I begin to lose sight of the new-

and-improved, stronger, wiser and humbler me.

Today is one of those days when I need to just keep the faith.

October 1, 2014

16 PRINCESS MARGARET HOSPITAL

When I used to hear the words Princess Margaret Hospital the first thing I'd think of was a home lottery. Everyone wanted to win one of the big prizes: the dream homes, the luxury cars, vacations and fun merchandise. I guess, like anyone else, I would've loved to win any of those too. But for some reason or another, I just never bought a ticket or knew anyone who ever won anything from that lottery before so I never bothered.

The next thing I thought about whenever I heard the name of the hospital was bad news. To me, Princess Margaret Hospital was a place where more often than not, people went to die. An end-of-life meeting place for those forced to face their mortality sooner than they hoped. "One of the top cancer research centers in the world", the literature that came in the mail used to say. Again, I used to simply glance over the brochures or skim the newspaper articles that shared patient survival stories at Princess Margaret Hospital.

Unconcerned and invincible would be how I'd describe my ambivalence towards all matters around cancer. The strange thing is my mother had died from an extremely rare and aggressive cancer so you'd think I'd have been hyper vigilant around these matters. *It's not going to happen to me,* I used to believe wholeheartedly. As an adult, I did whatever the articles and research studies told us we need to do to remain healthy and cancer-free. I used to exercise five times a week, I took vitamins daily, I drank cups of green tea everyday, I ate vegetables and fruit like a fiend, I didn't smoke and only had the occasional drink. No one in my mother's family had ever died from cancer so I thought her experience was exactly what we were told: a rare one-off, a one in five hundred thousand odd. It was a lottery that sadly, didn't work in her favor because she was the one who died too soon.

But on May 29, 2013 my husband pushed me in my wheelchair as we found our way around Princess Margaret Hospital for the first time. I remember looking around at the activity all around us. The blood lab was filled with patients of all ages, some bald and many not, waiting for their number to be called. The elevators were crammed with doctors in white coats, visitors carrying flowers and gifts, people like me in wheelchairs or walking with canes or walkers accompanied by their loved ones. I felt like I was in a busy airport or a mall around Christmas time, not a hospital. Being there in person, this place now felt like a meeting center, a place where people came to get answers, to find support and more than anything else, to hold onto hope.

While we were riding the glass elevators up to

the fourth floor that morning, I noticed a huge banner hanging down a long wall in the foyer that read: *"Princess Margaret Hospital . . . Believe. We will conquer cancer in our lifetime."* A hopeful and positive thing to read on your way to visit your oncologist for the first time. I found strength in those words and repeated them over and over in my head in the months to come.

If I had a feeling I was in the right place as we got off the elevator, then I definitely knew it two hours later when we got back on the elevator on our way out. From the warmth of voice from the nurse who escorted me to Dr. Krzyzanowska's examining room to the curious resident who came in and took down my history and conducted an examination on me, I felt like I was in great hands. But it was when Dr. Krzyzanowska entered the room and walked immediately over to meet me and shook my hand, when my body identified a feeling it had not felt in a long while: safety. Dr. Monika looked me straight in the eye and smiled. Her prognosis was hopeful. Her action plan for me seemed logical and thorough. She was going to follow me through. I never wanted to kiss a woman as much as I wanted to at that moment. *"Good news, finally"*, I texted to my sisters and close friends when Dr. Krzyzanowska stepped out of the room for a minute to grab something. Up until then, I had been sinking under the force of a tsunami and here was someone who was throwing me a life preserver. Princess Margaret Hospital was giving me hope.

Since that first visit I've been back to Princess Margaret regularly for CT scans, blood work, ultrasounds and various doctor appointments in order to continue with the close monitoring I require for early detection of any possible signs of disease. The truth is that whenever I enter the building, I feel lucky to be there in the hands of and under the watchful eyes of a team of very special specialists.

It feels like I've won a lottery after all.

October 7, 2014

17 WATER

It started with uncontrollable tears. Piles of used up tissues scattered across my bedroom floor when I'd wake up the next morning. I'd cry myself to sleep, whenever sleep came in those early days of the diagnosis. Those days when the information about what was wrong with me was incomplete, always-waiting more test results and doctor appointments.

The tears I shed were private in those early days, hidden from my husband and daughters. In the dark and quiet of one o'clock in the morning, after tossing and turning for a couple of hours, I'd leave my bed and go hide in our spare bedroom or head downstairs to the couch where I'd take up with another box of Kleenex. I cried out of fear. I cried from exhaustion. I cried whenever I pictured my eight and ten-year-old daughters' faces. I'd cry so hard I'd wake up with puffy eyes and a swollen complexion. I remember those nights of hell and wish them on nobody. Alone and scared, the crying eventually allowed my restless heart and erratic breathing to calm down. I'd wake up exhausted each day, after a night of crying, but my body somehow felt cleared of the emotional stress and sadness that had accumulated the day before. Looking back now, I credit those tears for giving me strength to face whatever was coming my way. The tears provided a release and taught me about my body's capacity to heal. My tears were, and still are, a lifeline. I cry a lot.

Months after my surgery (and immobility) and a few weeks after starting physiotherapy, the first steps I took towards active rehab were outside of my home and the physio table, but in my neighbor Kathy's pool. It was mid-September and

I remember my husband having to help me take the two or three steps into the shallow area of the pool. I remember submerging the two aluminum crutches into the water and they filling up with pool water. I managed to walk a few steps around the perimeter of the shallow end that day. The next day, I brought one of the pool noodles inside the pool with me and followed Sabrina's direction. I tried to press the noodle with my rehabiliating leg onto the pool floor. Back and forth I paced the area of Kathy's pool each day until the weather started to cool and I had to find someplace else to go.

Enter the hydrotherapy pool. Three times a week Carlo and I would go to a 94 degrees hot pool and there, I'd do basic exercises: kicks underwater, more stepping on noodles, standing on one leg at a time. After a couple of months of doing this, I tried to see if I could float again and I found some success. I was finally able to get both feet off the ground underwater; something I never thought I'd be able to do again.

Those first few floats eventually led to me completing one length of the pool swimming the front stroke. This time we were at a regular pool during a lane swim. While I had to endure the stares of swimmers watching me and staring at the twelve-inch scar down my thigh as I entered and exited the pool with my crutch, once immersed in water, I became like one of them again. I could swim. Slowly, at first, but after a few weeks, I managed to pick up speed. Floating horizontally in the water, I almost felt like my old self again except for my now heavier left leg dragging me down. I usually felt no pain. It was just me in swimmer's pose. Underwater, I was flooded with thoughts and memories of everything that I had gone through over those past few months. My rhythmic breaths soon began to feel not only familiar again but therapeutic as well. In and out my breath went, calming my muscles and slowing my thoughts.

What I couldn't realize back then but do now, was that all those lengths I swam back and forth were slowly propelling me forward and bringing the broken me back to life.

Following my swims, most days I'd make my way over to the hot tub. Whirling, hot water around me, I'd position my leg and hip joint strategically in front of the roaring jets to massage them after all their hard work. The hot tub forced me to slow down and wait for my muscles to respond in relaxation. Like meditation, being in the hot tub grounded me in the moment. There was nothing I could do but sit and wait and allow the forces around me to do what they needed to do. Submerged in the hot water, I surrendered and allowed the heat of the water to comfort my mind and my body. Even today at the new health club that I've recently joined, I continue to use the hot tub and steam room following my swims to ease pain, help me decompress and to continue to nurture myself back to health.

When I think about pain management this past year I picture my two go-to items. My hot water bottle and my Epsom salts baths (along with the occasional Tylenol and Arnica cream). Whether my quad muscles have been pinching or my calf muscle feels like it's on fire, I continue to turn to hot water to relieve me of pain. Nothing does the trick like a hot bath or a rest on the couch with my hot water bottle perched on my sore muscle.

Slowing down and allowing the warmth of the water to do what it needs to do that has taught me how healing can happen. Everyday I'm witness to the healing properties of water.

October 8, 2014

18 THE BIKE

I've always been a reader of memoirs. I enjoy learning about the life stories of others in the hopes of learning something about my own. I devour memoirs for any tidbit of wisdom or insight that sheds light for me in a way I never would've previously thought about.

One of my favorite memoirs was Lance Armstrong's *It's Not About the Bike: My Journey Back To Life*. This remarkable story about Armstrong's comeback from the darkest prospects of survival and recovery from brain, testicular and lung cancer was something I believed to be incredible. After my mother died from this disease, I never thought that a full recovery was possible for anyone. But not only did Armstrong miraculously recover from cancer, he went on to win a handful of Tour de France championships in the years that followed. Despite the revelations of his rampant use and denial of use of illegal steroids in the last few years and now that his hero ship is permanently tarnished, I still think about Lance's story every once in a while. In fact, I thought about it this morning as I stepped onto the indoor cycling bike at the health club before my spinning class began.

After several attempts at getting my seat's height adjusted properly and my handlebars positioned close enough for me to reach them without overextending my arms, I finally sat on the saddle and clicked my shoes into place on the pedals below. I gave my seat and handlebar settings a test run by spinning my pedals around for a few rotations to see if I felt comfortable. This elaborate ritual of getting on the bike and then getting off to adjust sometimes gets tiring, as it did this morning. I often wonder, like I did today, is it worth this . . . what am I doing here . . . I can't do this the way I want to. But I pushed aside that inner voice of doubt and got back on the seat and told myself "just one song . . . get through one song and then if you don't want to do this anymore, get off the bike". I pedaled through this morning's first song, "Walking On Sunshine", musing on the irony of the words walking and sunshine and imagining a healthy and energetic me walking, limp-free, along gigantic rays of sunshine. The song made me happy so I stayed on the bike for another one.

The next song initiated the beginning of many uphill climbs organized into the ride the instructor had planned for today. The task was to slowly and incrementally increase the tension on the bike's dial to mimic an uphill climb up a mountain. The higher we climbed, the harder it would get and the tighter our leg muscles would feel. The beauty of this climb was that everyone in the class was doing it but each of us at our own paces and in our own time. Although the other riders and I were in it together, we were ultimately riding alone. Like life, I thought.

The more I think about it, the more I realize that the rest of today's ride simulated life or at the very least was a poignant metaphor for it. It was the point Lance Armstrong was trying to make. At times, we pushed, and then pulled our way through. At others, we coasted but had to spin our way crazily back through other moments. We grasped the handlebars and held on for dear life while at other times we were able to let go and feel a little freer. Some of us broke a sweat while others of us glowed. A few of us made the ride look easy while others wore the struggle of the climb all over our faces. I looked around at all of us, men and women alike, of various ages, shapes and sizes, each bearing an assortment of aches and pains climbing our own hills and was reminded of a quote I had recently read in the morning paper.

"Hills are our friends. The challenges in our lives become easier the more we face them. Hills become easier the more that you run them."

If I were to look at this recovery I'm on in terms of being one gigantic hill, I wonder where I am on the mountain. Are my challenges getting easier the more I face them? *Easier?* A word I'd never choose to describe recovery.

October 16, 2014

19 DREAMS

In my dreams, I'm walking normally. Without a limp, an ache or a pause in step, I walk. In my dreams, I watch myself walk and notice exactly how I'm walking. And that's what I remember most when I wake up from the dream. The *how*. I've been keeping a dream journal for years where I record my dreams. Here are a few of them.

In one of my recent dreams, I was carrying a baby of about nine or ten months in my arms. I recall how I was actually carrying and walking the baby around on my own two feet. This exhilarated me. A weak leg and a prominent limp is not the safest vessel in which a parent would want their child to be carried. So since my once-strong leg has been taken away from me I haven't held and carried an infant in a standing position, let alone moving with one in my arms. No longer do I sway back and forth or pace up and down carrying a baby like I used to love to do when my daughters were babies. It's felt like another of life's little joys snatched away from me. To have someone so soft and little and lovable trust you to hold him or her safely is one of the best feelings I know. And to no longer be able to be able to do that is saddening for me, a deep loss. So when, in that dream, I was walking limp–free, and holding an infant, I woke up feeling like I'd actually been soaring.

Another dream I had earlier in the spring of this year was of me, post-surgery and post-recovery, jogging once again in our neighborhood like I used to do. In my dream, as I was jogging, I was looking down at both of my legs, shaking my head in disbelief saying to myself, "Dr. Wunder said I'd never run again and look at me." I remember that, in the dream, I had had no pain at all while running, like I used to. Both in the dream and once I'd awaken from it, I felt elated. In fact, as I now read my dream journal where I recorded this dream back on May 29th of this year, I wrote the words "I'm on Cloud Nine" at the end of the entry.

Just a few weeks ago I had recorded this particular entry in my dream journal: *In last night's dream, I was watching myself and had a moment. I was wearing heels for the first time! They were black booties with a one-inch heel. The feeling I've woken up with is absolute surprise . . . pride, even.* Surprise and pride. I'd say happiness would be another.

But then I thumb through earlier dream entries and stop at the April 14th one where I describe having dreamed of water freezing around me. In it, I'm carefully trying to avoid walking over frozen patches of water. I'm scared of slipping on the ice both on foot and driving my car. My entry reads: *Over and over again, throughout the dream, I'm avoiding the slippery and frozen parts.* After this one, I remember waking up feeling fearful and unsettled.

Thoughts of my mobility, or lack thereof, seem to be at the forefront of my mind. When I'm watching tv or a movie, I study the way the actors move freely and without second thought. When I'm at the health club or sitting on a park bench I watch others move about around me and wonder if I'll ever stroll again or be able to pick up a towel that I've dropped without other people staring at me. If I walk in a shoe store, I always stop for an extra second or two to admire the high-heeled shoes and question whether I'll ever slip my feet into a pair again. More mourning. Another loss. Not a huge loss on the scale of losses but something I miss just the same.

I sometimes wonder if all this observing that I do, of able and moving bodies around me, and all the grieving that I go through everyday at the loss of some of my mobility seeps into my subconscious and then releases itself at night in my dreams. My daytime obsessions around my current recovery process and my speculations around how much better, worse, or the same I'll be able to walk in a few years' time seem to be playing themselves out in my dreams. The walking that I do in my dreams is both metaphorical and literal. In these nighttime visions, the icy patches that I avoid or the high heels that I prance around in with glee seem to reflect my general sense of emotional wellbeing at that time. Some days I'm hopeful for a successful recovery and a return to many of the things I was able to do before, like travelling on foot more or standing for longer periods of time without tiring. Other days I feel scared of what may lie ahead. A return of the cancer and another frightening journey down that icy road.

My dreams feel like unsolved puzzles. But what I'm learning is that when I wake up and feel the need to quickly record them before I lose sight of them in my mind, I should pay attention.

How I feel when I wake up is a sign that I'm fully alive.

I'm going to end this now so I can take advantage of this glorious fall day and go outside for a walk, poles and all.

October 22, 2014

20 INSPIRATION

"Do you mind if I ask what happened to you?" asked the young guy working behind the counter at the café inside the health club I go to. The question, for some reason, caught me off guard. I mean I'm used to the curious looks and the odd question asked but this guy seemed really curious. He really wanted to know.

"It's just that . . . I see you come in here everyday . . . and you look like you're in pain . . ." he added. And so, while paying for a protein bar I was hoping to gobble down before my spinning class was to begin, I gave him the brief, bulleted version of my story: cancerous tumor growing on top of the femur, femur had to be cut off, prostheses in place, major muscles group cut out, will walk with a limp forever. Done. I retold the story and was relieved that today it came out easier than normal. Easier, that is, until the young man said those three words that make me cringe.

"You're an inspiration," he said. No! I don't feel like an inspiration, I thought to myself but didn't say out loud. Instead, I nodded to him and then quickly hobbled away before tears surfaced. I made it inside the change room and then had my good cry inside the washroom stall.

The rest of that day was what I call a downer. Although I did manage to get to the spinning class, afterwards I couldn't get myself off the couch. Self-pity came to join me and so did anger. How did this happen to me? Anger had spoken up: *I don't want to be anyone's inspiration* . . . I want my leg back. Self-pity got her two cents in as well: *Why me?* It was Anger's volley: *I'm always going to be disabled.* It was self-pity's turn. Back and forth the two of them bantered, leaving me a little more worse for wear emotionally at the end of the day than I had been at the start.

But I've been thinking about this idea of me being an inspiration to others a lot more since this happened. In fact, just yesterday it happened again. I was leaving my friend's place after having tea when I told her that I needed to sit down somewhere in order to put on my boots (I can't reach my left foot from a standing position). And as I was bending over and struggling to reach the zipper on my boot, she said it.

"Gina, you're an inspiration."

"Oh," I said, "I hate when people say that. I don't feel in any way inspiring."

"Oh, okay," she said," I won't say that anymore." She's a sweet person who meant well. I immediately felt terrible for saying what I did, however truthful I was being.

So why do I feel so uncomfortable when someone calls me inspiring? Why do I feel like crying when people say to me "you've been through a lot"?

I've always believed that having empathy towards others is a gift. Whoever can put themselves in someone else's shoes and try to imagine feeling how that other person might be feeling has one of life's most important life skills. I've always been drawn to empathetic people. I tend to like people who seek to understand others instead of judging them. Maybe I got this from my mother who was empathic to a fault. She was a bona fide sucker for the underdog, a friend to the proverbial leper. My sisters and I had to have inherited this from her. And so if I think about the phrase "you're an inspiration, Gina" from this viewpoint, of the empathetic, I feel honored that others are imagining the difficulties I've endured and continue to acknowledge it with those three words. We're all one.

But many times for me, being the *object* of another's empathy or inspiration feels unwanted, especially when I wake up everyday wishing my reality could be different. When others' commend me for handling this struggle that I've been dealt, inside I feel very isolated and alone. If they refer to my strength, both inner and outer, I feel weak. How can I inspire others when deep down inside I feel so sad about and unaccepting of my disabled body? I feel like a fraud. How can I inspire able-bodied people who are physically capable of doing a lot more than I can do? They're the lucky ones, I'm not, I know. By looking at me, do they feel inspired to not complain when they have a sore back that will go away or a minor running injury? Or, do I remind people of the fragility of life and how it takes only an instant for your life to be turned upside down? Does that inspire them to live more honestly and gratefully? I've no idea. Maybe I should ask them next time.

So if I want to somehow turn lemons into lemonade and finally feel deserving of the praise I receive for being an inspiration to others, what must I do? Here is the list of answers I've come up with so far based on how I've been living my life since the cancer arrived on my lemonade stand. Keep carrying on, don't stop, and try not to complain, hold onto hope, never give up and strive to have the life experiences that I've always wanted to have despite this battered leg of mine.

November 19, 2014

21 CARLY AND ME

In early January of 2013, fresh off the heels of writing and self-publishing my first novel, a burst of creative energy came to me and I knew that I wanted to start writing my next book immediately. With my kids at an independent age and a recent shift in my career happily underway, I had finally taken up the hobby I had always promised myself that I'd get to one day: writing. The fact that I managed to write in the early hours of every morning, sometimes squeezing in my morning swim beforehand, confirmed a solid commitment to this venture on my part.

So it was on one of those dark, cold January mornings as I was driving out of the parking lot of the pool when a vision started to come to me.

My next character was beginning to introduce herself. And in my mind's eye, who I saw was a young woman, in her early to mid-twenties, attractive, tall and athletic. But with the zoom lens of my eye's camera, I focused in more closely on her face. And I saw the scar. My character would have a deep, horizontal scar about five inches wide running just above her brow line. I knew that it was a permanent one.

In the days that followed I wondered about my new character. For one, how did she get the scar? Two, how did she face her world everyday when she felt repulsed by the image staring back at her in the mirror? Scars are evidence of battle, I believed. Of what horror did that image in the mirror remind her? Three, I thought back to when I was in my twenties and how important feeling attractive felt to me so I wondered how this character navigated through the dating scene, if at all. With these questions and a few more in mind, I set out to get to know my character and her story in the weeks to come. Quite ironically, somewhere along the way, my character Carly's story began to run parallel with my own.

In early February of that year, I started to visit a sports' chiropractor for a recent limp in my step that I'd been experiencing and the feeling of there being something deep in my groin. This chiropractor also happened to be my first cousin, Carm. In his hands, I lay at his mercy to manipulate my joints and treat what I had thought to be a running injury. On his table, I took the opportunity to ask him questions about car accident injuries.

Throughout the three weeks or so that I visited him, our conversations in the treatment room often turned to Carly, my newly named protagonist. By this point, I knew that Carly had been in a horrific car accident but I needed to understand the impact a head-on car crash would have on her body, and more specifically, on the bones in her body. I remember the day I asked him about the femur: is it possible for the femur to break and how bad must the impact be in order to do so? Could both femurs break? Would surgery be necessary to repair these breaks? What would recovery be like? Then one day I asked him how someone could possibly end up with a permanent horizontal scar above the brow line as a result of a head-on collision.

"Easy," he answered as he was inserting acupuncture needles along my hip and groin areas, "glasses. Her glasses would lift up and get crushed by air bags . . . if the impact was fast and hard enough." There. I had it. So I began to write Carly's story.

Every morning for the next month and a half, I'd wake up and write drafts of early chapters. Scarred and traumatized from a terrible car accident that she herself had caused a few years earlier, Carly was now drowning in guilt from the lies she had told surrounding the accident. She was ashamed of the scar on her face and everyday covered it meticulously with products and makeup. Carly was trying to build a new life for herself post-recovery by returning to school to become an auto engineer and paying for it with her income from her part-time position in car sales. She may have been keeping her secrets about what really caused the crash but she was carrying around the shame those secrets caused her in the form of her scar.

So Carly's story was beginning to take shape in my mind and on my computer. That is, until the morning of Tuesday, March 19th. I had skipped out on writing that morning due to an appointment I had scheduled with Carm. He was to be giving me the results of the recent MRI I had undergone the week before.

"You have a mass," Carm began. "It's a bone tumour, Gi. And it's sitting on top of your left femur."

The next time I opened my Carly Book file (what I used to call my early drafts) was late May.

In the two and half months in between, my own life had been upended by the terror of a cancer diagnosis and a long search for answers about the rare type and location of the cancer I had. In that time, I'd been operated on twice, had been told not to place any weight on my left leg whatsoever, was mobile only with the use of a walker, crutches and wheelchair, had visited top specialists at two hospitals who had ordered extensive medical tests that I had to go through. I was holding onto dear life with every muscle of my being.

So while still waiting for test results and further direction from my oncologists, I sat at my dining room table that sunny day and decided to get reacquainted with Carly again. I'm not quite sure what brought me to my laptop that day. I was pretty certain that I wouldn't be able to concentrate on writing. But something happened as I was opening the file. I realized that I knew Carly a lot better. I understood her loss of physical freedom, her struggle with mobility, and the shock of her life changing in an instant. I could follow her struggle better because I was experiencing loss, mobility issues and hardest of all, trauma of my own.

In the months to come, I would write about Carly's post-surgical recovery as I was enduring my own. I'd recount her feelings of depression and isolation as I was experiencing them myself. On days when I was feeling hopeful, Carly's thoughts would be more positive. On my darker days, Carly seemed to understand and somehow helped pull me through. And although Carly's story eventually took turns that my own life wasn't taking, I'm not sure she would've arrived at her place of self-forgiveness and acceptance had I not been on a difficult journey of my own.

All of this makes me wonder now, months after my Carly book has been finished and published, how in control I had thought I was of my story in those early winter months before my diagnosis? There I was seeking answers from experts in order to create a believable story about someone's struggle but little did I know that I'd become the most ironic expert of all. I'm also curious, as I massage the twelve and half inch scar that runs along my outer left thigh and hip area, about the vision that came to me that morning of that physically and emotionally scarred girl. Was she foreshadowing the battle that lay ahead for me? My own scar wonders.

November 20, 2014

.

22 DISCARD PILE

1. Favorite purple V-neck cashmere sweater

2. Once-worn studded salmon-colored blouse

3. Short sleeve white cotton eyelet blouse

4. Relatively new tan blouse with rope tassels

5. Black Speedo training suit

6. Size eight suede high-heeled sandals

7. Approximately five other pairs of shoes with higher-than-half-inch heels, wedges or no grip on the sole

8. Slippers that I wore in the hospital

All of these items went straight to the trash. As I came across each article in my closet, I either yanked it off its' hanger or pulled them out of the shoeboxes and immediately threw in a discard pile. Whether it was relatively new and not worn much or was a wardrobe staple that I'd grown attached to didn't matter. Each piece marked an inerasable moment in my journey and sparked a negative memory. It had to go. I knew I could never wear any of these things again and not recall the time I wore it last: inside a doctor's office receiving unwanted news, getting out of the hospital bed for the first time following my three surgeries, remembering how much I loved to wear wedges and knowing that I'd likely never be able to again. All of these items brought me pain. They reminded me of everything I had lost.

Today I open my closet doors and take pride in my new wardrobe of yoga pants, sweat socks, Roots sweaters, workout tanks, cycling shoes and updated Speedo bathing suits. These, I tell myself, are the clothes of recovery. I wear them everyday to the health club, to my physiotherapy appointments, and on walks around the neighborhood with my walking poles. These clothes make me happy. Wearing them, I'm motivated to keep working at the job I have to do: walking again unaided, building muscle, getting stronger. Psychologically, they help me build confidence in myself. When I look in the mirror while wearing them I don't see the disabled me: crooked, weak, unfit and disabled. Some days, these clothes even help me feel like a little more like my old, fitter self again.

If I take a step back (in my flat boots) and try to look at the big picture, what I see is that my clothes, like my music and my writing, are helping me to interpret my new reality. They bring me back into the present when my mind wants to wander into the future or dwell in the past. Here I am right now at home washing a load of workout wear that I wore all week at the gym. My mantra comes to me: all I have is today. *Wear* your present moment.

Another thought comes to me: I'm alive and "living" in my clothes and so grateful.

November 28, 2014

23 THE QUOTE

People have asked me how I've gotten through everything that I have had to. *If they only knew the half of it* is the first thing that comes to mind. The reason I say this is because I really don't know what these people are referring to specifically. I've been through a lot. I've been through more than most people think I've been through. And I'm still going through heavy stuff. I know that I will be for the rest of my life.

So, are these people wondering how I got through the scare of the cancer diagnosis? Or are they imagining the nightmare of having three five to eight-hour surgeries in a two-month span? Or, when they see me wobble, limp, or look like I'm in pain, are they empathizing with my loss of mobility? I never know where the question is coming from so I don't say much.

Instead I turn inward and recite to myself the quote I had found a while ago but can't recall where I found it. It may have been on one of those Internet quotation sites or in a book I read. I just remember writing it down. It's a quote that, as soon as I had read it, felt was written for me. Gently, it whispers to me to surrender and let go. And while I'm reading the quote, I do just that. I see a great big question mark forming in my mind and, as foreign as it feels, I embrace it. The quote may not be an obvious response to the question of how I've gotten through this difficult time, but for me, it helps me recognize the strategy that is working for me: acceptance.

This is the Joseph Campbell quote that's posted next to my laptop . . . and in my brain.

"We must let go of the life we have planned, so as to accept the one that is waiting for us."

I'm trying.

December 3, 2014

24 WORK IN PROGRESS

Usually after I've written one of these reflections, I make myself wait a couple of weeks or longer before allowing myself to reread it. I do this for a couple of reasons. One, I'm interested in my progress or lack thereof. I don't necessarily mean my physical progress such as tracking my pain (more, less or about the same) or my leg strength (more, less or more of the same). What I'm referring to is my emotional and psychological states of mind. For example, in rereading the entries I try to gauge the mood I was in on the day I'd written these entries. Was I hopeful . . . bored . . . frustrated . . . feeling lost? Or, I look for what, if anything, have I learned about this journey that I'm on? I also search for clues in my writing that indicate that perhaps I am moving past my fears. No surprise that I get disappointed when the evidence comes out minimal or insufficient sometimes. *Be kind to yourself,* I remind myself. Aren't I writing to work my way through this? I desperately want to get better in every way, that inevitably, my patience runs thin and I begin to lose hope. I'm never going to walk without this horrible limp, or I feel so alone and scared when I think of the future. These are typical impatient thoughts for me.

Another reason why I wait before rereading past entries is because I'm hoping that the passage of time in between writing and reading the pieces will highlight the honesty in which I write. I'm looking for a theme to emerge or a thread to be woven. Whether I'm going to publish these entries for public reading (such as in a book, blog, or essay contest entries) or not is still up in the air, I try to step back and read these pieces as a reader instead of the writer. Would I pick up a book about this woman's experiences? Am I curious enough to learn about her story? Does the reader in me connect with this author's writing style? Would I be able to see myself at all in her story and if not, would I still be interested in reading about it?

I suppose these all sound like "editor-type" questions but at a deeper level I suppose I'm trying to determine if I have a story at all. Everyone has a story . . . this is yours. Yes, I know this is true on an intellectual level. But when I turn the lens from writer to reader I worry that, collectively, my entries might be weighing a bit too heavily on the . . . *heavy* and that I'll lose my reader in the midst of it all. I can see someone shaking his head and thinking *isn't she just grateful to be alive?* Or I hear a critical reader in my midst asking *what's this author point* and closing the book with a big, loud thud.

I sit on this last thought for a while. I always do. And while I acknowledge that the actual act of writing these entries has been therapeutic for me, I'm still not convinced that reading about them, although honest and linear in their progression, are relatable or relevant or interesting enough.

This, like me, is definitely a work in progress. Sigh.

December 11, 2014

25 FICTIONAL FRIENDS

Downton Abbey made me cry.

Homeland gripped me and never let me go.

Call The Midwife allowed me to grieve.

Girls was a guilty distraction.

Veep was entertaining.

Masters Of Sex was like fine literature . . . rich and satisfying.

The Affair made me think (but not about having an affair).

The Fall scared the life out of me but I couldn't stop watching.

Both *Hostages* and *Stalker* made me swoon . . . over Dylan McDermott.

How To Get Away With Murder was the one that I shared with my husband.

The Returned infuriated me.

Game Of Thrones saved me.

All of these TV shows came into my life at a time when I felt that I was losing control of it. Hurled onto to the couch against my wishes, I was stuck, literally and figuratively. "No weight-bearing on your left leg whatsoever," Dr. Wunder and his team told me over and again following my first two biopsies. They sent me home from hospital with instructions. I could do nothing but wait for direction from them as to my next steps (pun intended). And so, my life of limited mobility had begun.

But surprising to me, so too did my relationship with a group of fascinating fictional television characters that never would have otherwise come to me. Before the cancer, I had always been a reader. My idea of relaxing after a long day's work was to lie in bed and read. Sometimes, the odd sitcom would steal my attention but I wasn't invested in any one series.

To me, TV watching was a waste of precious time that I, a full-time working mother, felt was in dwindling supply.

The Crawleys, though, drew me in like a magnet. Everyday, I found myself anxious to listen to the sound of the delicate piano keys playing in the *Downton Abbey* opening theme. Strategically, I'd ration each episode, watching only one a day. How I wanted them to last! Lying on that couch with my laptop propped up beside me, I'd escape into a completely different world similar to the one I inhabited whenever I read. But at this time of turmoil in my own life I was having a hard time concentrating on reading fiction so to watch it unfold in front of me onscreen was exactly what I needed. These shows offered me an escape and I took it.

Living with the unknown, as I was doing at that time, as well as being humbled by my recently shaken world, I had begun to relate to the characters in these shows in a way I had never been able to before. These characters' storylines and dramas revealed themes that were now resonating with me. I remember one line that Mrs. Hughes said in one of the early *Downton Abbey* seasons. "You only ever have one mother, don't you?" she asked after one of the character's had lost his mother. I remember pausing the computer, grabbing a pen and writing that line down. It was poetry to my ears. That single line reopened the gates to my grieving world, allowing me to feel my loss over again.

On the opposite side of death is life, which is what I was reminded of after each episode of *Call The Midwife*. There, in late 1950s inner city London, England, midwives were called to deliver life, full of tragedies and joys and complications. I remember one episode when a mother delivered a baby boy who was slightly deformed and later found to have spina bifida. The heartbroken mother blamed herself for the baby's misfortune and then avoided the baby by denying him her love and attention. For the mother, life didn't turn out the way it was supposed to, a theme I too was living and relating with.

I can go on talking about these shows as if I was an entertainment critic but what I love most about watching all them is sharing them with others. Whether I'm debriefing *The Affair* with my sister Daniela or crushing over Jon Snow in *Game of Thrones* with Jenn or Pina, I know that as soon as I finish watching the episode I have these people to call, text, email or send some online article related to that particular episode. While I read the discussion boards and follow the discourse on these shows in cyberspace, there is nothing like hearing my friends' opinions on these characters and stories and us having a good laugh over them. I feel like I'm a part of many exclusive book clubs with different members. We connect post-episode airing, where no spoiler alerts need to be issued and trashing is more than allowed.

So what I've learned is that for me, the best thing to do sometimes is to just get out of my thinking, worrying, imagining, analyzing head. These shows let me do that. They have been and continue to be the perfect distraction. Which is why I say that at the toughest parts of my journey, they saved me.

December 22, 2014

26 EARLY CHRISTMAS GIFT

This morning I got a surprising and early Christmas gift. It didn't occur to me at first that it was even happening. I sat down on my chair in the dressing area of my bedroom, as I do every morning. I threw my scrunched up sock on the floor in front of me as I usually do. Then the toes of my left foot began to crawl into the waiting sock as they always do. Since the surgery, I haven't been able to reach down to put on my own sock. I can't clip my toenails or shave my left shin either. I get stuck somewhere along the way. My hands can no longer reach their destination and then I have no choice but to give up. Thank goodness for frequent visits to get a pedicure and for laser hair removal, which have removed two of these obstacles for me. But putting on socks and tying shoes still escape me. That is, until this morning.

Without even realizing I was doing it until after it was done, fingers on my right hand had reached down and scooped the sock from beneath my left foot and pulled it all the way around my heel. And in one swoop my sock was on. Whoa! Once the shock had subsided, pure joy had seeped through. It took eighteen months of post-surgery recovery and waiting but it finally happened. The impossible was actually possible. Putting on a sock? Who would have ever thought it could be so . . . awesome.

The second part of my gift came a little later at the gym. It's Tuesday. The day I do machines, weights and floor exercises. I had removed my winter boots when I got to the locker and started changing into my runners. This usually is a process that involves tying the left shoe's laces on my lap first and then throwing the shoe on the floor and letting my toes make their way inside the shoe. Then, the shoehorn comes out of my gym bag, like a rabbit out of a hat, and the magic happens. Presto. Shoe on left foot. If my laces for some reason become untied . . . you guessed it, the whole process starts again.

But today, both of my hands reached the laces. I watched as my fingers managed to tie them together in a knot. JOY. Then astonishment. I grabbed my phone, fumbling with excitement, and took a picture of one of my hands reaching the laces. Then I pressed the 'video' button on my phone and tried to capture it 'live'. It was as if it was the birth of a baby or an Olympic performance of some kind, a once–in a lifetime that can't be missed. But seeing how I needed both hands to tie a shoelace and one of them was holding a phone, the video of the miracle lace-tying event didn't exactly work.

So, here comes the dramatic overture. Cue the music, please. It feels like Christmas came a little earlier for me this year and I got the most unexpected but wonderful gift: a sign that I'm making progress.

December 23, 2014

27 THE PARKING PERMIT

Everyday it feels like I experience some sort of discrimination separate from my disability. I'm not sure what to call it though. Ageism? No, that's not it although I think it might have something to do with it. Maybe it's not discrimination that I'm feeling as much as an uncomfortable and frustrating sense of presumption of guilty behavior? It happens to me so often, at least a few times a day that it's now beginning to make me just a little bit angry.

It's the parking permit that I use whenever I pull into a parking space reserved for handicapped persons. I'm a legitimate user of the permit. Whether I'm at the gym or the library, a shopping plaza or a doctor's office I can never seem to pull into the spot without getting the glares and stares of onlookers. What I've noticed is that more times than not, people out there are watching. I call them the benevolent handicap parking space watchers, ready to pounce on any offender who slips into one of these spots even for a quick two-minute errand they need to run. For this, I appreciate their vigilance because these spots are few and far between and there are many of us who really need them. Calling on someone who has parked in one of these spots and who doesn't have a parking pass visible on their windshield is the right thing to do. Public shaming does work. So, thank you for guarding what is ours to use and for speaking up against the ignorant and selfish who try to take advantage of something they (luckily) have no right to.

But my frustration rises from the looks *I* get when I'm pulling into a spot and my pass is clearly visible. I've gotten the stare-down where the passerby holds his/her stare until I'm parked and then waits for me to get out of my vehicle. It's as if he or she is watching to make sure I'm legit. And when I pull out my cane and slowly roll out of my seat, they look away. Sometimes. Because this stare-down happens so often, I've begun a little ritual where I hold up my parking permit facing outward while I'm driving into the parking lot heading for the handicap spots. I'm flashing my sign for all to see. Then, once parked, I place the sign on the windshield and begin my exit out of my vehicle. The other thing I do is I take my cane with me even for quick stops or if the entrance is close enough and I'd normally leave my cane in the car. It's like I have to prove my legitimacy with the use of my cane. And this is what rattles me a bit.

It's the judgments we make based on looks, stereotypes and impressions. When we think of handicap parking space users we typically picture the aged either hunched over, limping, walking at a snail's pace or paralyzed altogether. We don't picture forty plus year old longhaired brunettes with makeup and sunglasses on. If we see one of these women pull into a handicap spot we assume she's a busy soccer mom, in a hurry, using the closest available parking space to run her errand. Or, we think she's taking advantage of using the pass that belongs to her parent and doesn't really need the parking space for herself. And if, at first glance, she exits her car and seems to look fine and normal we call her on it. Guilty! I know because this has happened to me twice since I've started using the parking pass. And both times I felt this burning rage build inside me.

Damn it! Do you think I want to use this parking space? I'd do anything to park in the farthest spot in this whole (expletive) lot if I could.

Mind your own (expletive) business!

I'm bloody disabled! Can't you see that?

Wanna trade places?

Why do I have to defend myself here?

All of these thoughts have crossed my mind

but haven't come out of my mouth. Instead, I reply with no words. I wave my cane in the air and walk away. Words don't escape me. Instead, anger sets in for a while until I decide to let it go.

Until tomorrow, that is, when I'm sure it'll happen again.

January 5, 2015

28 LESSONS IN SHORTSIGHTEDNESS

I'm at the point in my recovery, I think, when I'm starting to ask myself how did I get here? The shortsightedness that I was suffering from for the longest time, that inability to see the bigger picture, is starting to fade. Convinced that I was never going to walk again without an aid or that my life was only going to ever be about doctor appointments and medical tests were ways I was completely blind to the possibility that in time, things change. When after a year post-surgery I was still suffering from depression and experiencing post-traumatic stress symptoms almost on a daily basis I had concluded that this was my new life and the sooner I accepted it, the better.

The funny thing is that when I started identifying myself as disabled and when I tried to make peace with the fact that I can no longer do some of the things I used to love to do is when I started to feel better and things started to change. Emotionally and physically it was like I had been stuck, unaccepting of my reality, that held back my progress. Yes, I am still walking with a cane and limping around like a wounded war vet but my energy is improving and hope is starting to make a humble homecoming. Can I do stairs yet? Not even close, but that's all right. I'll keep working at it. But am I able to bend down and pick up a piece of paper that I've dropped? Better than I could a few months ago.

For some reason, last night I was thinking about my time in the dark place, those long months when I felt so alone and couldn't see my way out. I remember my therapist telling me to imagine myself trudging through this dark forest with only a lantern in my hand, not a flashlight, guiding me. One step at a time was the only way out because that's as far as I could see. Taking each step was painful in more ways than just the obvious. But I took the one step even in the dimmest light.

The imagery of the forest and the lantern came at a perfect time. I found these images comforting because during this time I'd been trying so hard to see a way out of that forest but couldn't. I'd wake up everyday with the same heavy leg pounding on the floor on the way to the bathroom and fatigue would wash over me. *I don't want to do this anymore. I want my old leg back. Not another day of this,* I used to think, *when is this ever going to get better . . . easier?* I was crying for the future ahead of me and I was mourning the past behind me. I was living in a present that brought me little comfort because the present was hellish. So with no other choice in front of me, I decided to take Janice's advice. I picked up the proverbial lantern and I surrendered myself to the darkness.

This was the best lesson in shortsightedness so far. Let go but hang on.

January 15, 2015

29 OTHERS WHO'VE BEEN THERE

Thanks to email, I've connected with a few people who've been *there*. By there, I mean, the places where never in a million years we'd have ever thought we'd be one day, on the receiving end of a frightening diagnosis. I've talked a lot about feeling alone and in the dark throughout those months following my surgery. I really was never alone physically, surrounded by the love and attention of my husband, my children, my sisters, my godmother, friends, my in-laws, my cousins, and neighbors. I felt nothing but love and patience and positive vibes from all of these people around me.

But even in this home full of supporters, feelings of isolation and depression still plagued me. I remember yearning to talk to someone who could relate in any way to the hell I was in. I suppose I was hoping to find someone who'd tell me the words I was hoping to hear: *"you'll get better"* or *"it gets harder before it gets easier"*. Or even, "it was like that for me, too."

I came to connect, throughout that first year of my recovery, with a few people who were able to say those words that I wanted to hear. After scouring the web and coming up empty with people who either blogged, Facebooked, Tweeted, or spoke about recovering from a similar trauma as mine, I turned to my surgeon at my three month post-op checkup and asked him if he could help connect me with anyone I could talk to about how I was feeling. He did.

Enter Melissa T. A young nurse living five hours away in North Bay, Ontario who travels down to Toronto every three months for visits with our doctor, Dr. Wunder. When she emailed me from the waiting room the day that Dr.

Wunder had asked her if she'd mind speaking to me, I knew the universe had answered my call for help. Dozens of emails and text messages followed and still continue to until this day. Although our stages in life and circumstances are different and our surgeries overlapped in only some ways, being in touch with Melissa, a fellow survivor, I believe has contributed to my recovery. When doubt grips me like a vice or when fear paralyzes me, I grab my device and contact Melissa. She responds in seconds (not exaggerating). More times than not, she manages to calm me down even by something as simple as reminding me that she used to feel what I'm feeling now. And then I feel better. Having Melissa has made me feel less alone on the darker days and having Melissa makes me feel even more triumphant on my stronger days because I can share them with her.

Here are snippets of some emails that she had sent me back in November of 2013, about a month after we connected.

I promise you the emotional stuff will get easier. You should soon be able to look back and realize how far you have come.

I had to keep pushing in order to get where I am now.

Another person I came in contact with in July of 2014 was Alfaan. I had read a Toronto Star article about a young man who had survived a grueling 28 hour surgery to remove a tumor near his spine that had grown to the size of a medium Tim Hortons' cup (that was the headline in the Toronto Star). In the article, the reporter had quoted Alfaan talking about his hard and long recovery. After reading the article several times, I knew I needed to talk to him. So I contacted the reporter and she agreed to set me up with Alfaan via email. Although Alfaan and I only exchanged one email, I feel his message to me came at a time when my faith in getting better was dwindling. Here are a couple of parts of his response that helped me.

Let me start by saying I'm not a hero. I'm just a regular guy that had cancer and I'm determined to fight it to the finish.

Next time we talk you'll be the hero I talk about.

Connecting with these strangers who didn't know me but probably understood me better at that time in my life than anyone made my journey through the dark less lonely. I clung to Melissa and Alfaan's words as tightly as I did to the small invisible lantern in my hand guiding me through the darkness. Maybe it's because I've always found solace in words: written, spoken, sung, read. Maybe it's because their experiences made me feel like mine were something I would and could get through. Maybe it was simply the connection with other that I was craving on a deeper level. Maybe it's all of these things and more or none of them at all.

I'm as grateful for the two of them as I am for everyone else in my life who's been here to help me.

January 25, 2015

30 FEBRUARY 2015

February 2015 goes down as being Toronto's coldest month on record. And we survived it. I didn't write a single reflection throughout the entire month, the longest I've gone so far without chronicling my journey. Here is what I did instead.

Out of twenty-eight days in February, I went to the gym twenty-two of them. I filled many days with appointments. I saw my physiotherapist twice. I had a massage treatment. I booked a one-hour session in the Aqua-Ciser with a personal trainer at the gym. He worked me so hard I was sore for days. I went to the hair salon for a color. Earlier in the month I met two friends for a quick lunch at Subway. I continued to work my way through an online course submitting assignments by their deadlines and posting responses almost daily on the discussion boards. Attending a bridal shower, reading four books (one of them was *The Girl on The Train*) and watching a few television series online also filled the time. My friend Lil and I met for pancakes at Cora's on Pancake Tuesday. My daughter Annabel performed at a Kiwanis festival with her school band so I went to support her. I continued to accompany my younger daughter Karina to her weekly ball hockey games. And towards the end of the month, I decided to spend some time each day writing short stories. I'm still editing the three I completed.

I thought about writing a reflection but I couldn't. Because in the midst of all these activities, I was also experiencing severe PTSD symptoms, and writing about them while they were happening seemed impossible to do. A thought, an odd symptom or upcoming dates for a medical appointment seem to be my PTSD triggers. And if time allows me to perseverate on any of these, then my PTSD kicks into high gear. In my case, it was a feeling of lightheadedness one day followed by a dizzy spell that set the ball in motion and for the next three weeks I was a mess emotionally and mentally. What caused the spell I'm not sure. But I know that afterwards a barrage of irrational thoughts flooded in followed by uncontrollable fear, my typical pattern. The fear triggered immobilization and isolation. *If I just lie on the couch and don't talk about it then maybe it isn't happening,* I thought. I told no one what I was going through but my husband could see I was in that state again. Panic and worry consumed me. Is the cancer coming back? Am I going to make it? So in between visits to the gym and reading books and writing stories about characters I was trying to get to know, my mind and body were fighting off those familiar feelings of fear, sorrow, and angst. The times I kept busy with outings and watching television were a reprieve from the craziness. As soon as I was alone with my thoughts again, the symptoms would return.

Some days, I managed to jot down thoughts in my journal and record physical symptoms that I was feeling. Putting pen to paper during this time was a challenge in itself. Looking back now, I wonder whether I had written about my difficult day while I was in the midst of having one would've comforted me. But I'm not sure how it could've because as I was going through it, I remember feeling that words were inaccessible to me. PTSD swept me away into this other world far away from logic, calm, and safety. It was a long and cold month. So when writing as therapy, one of my strongest lifelines, was unreachable to me I turned to another, my therapist Janice.

"You need to be held, Gina," Janice said, "Someone needs to hold you."

I made one other appointment in February. For the first time ever, I visited a craniosacral therapist. And I was held. I thank Nadine, this therapist with a special kind of touch, for joining me on my healing journey exactly when I needed her. The work of getting me to walk again had been looked after by my doctors and physio and massage therapists by this point but for the work of deeper emotional healing, I need Nadine.

March 3, 2015

31 IN LOVE WITH MY RADIO

I have recently undertaken a love affair with my radio. Lately, nothing has taken me out of my head better than this thing. My subscription to satellite radio has been my savior and my teacher. Like a lover, I'm devoted to it. I organize my days driving around town at the times my favorite programs air in the satellite radio in my car. At night, I sneak out into my car in the driveway and listen to segments that I missed earlier in the day that are re-airing. If I don't drive anywhere for a few days, I miss the enticement of the XM radio and feel like I've abandoned it. Of course I could buy another radio and a subscription for my house and listen to it all day but then the allure would be lost.

Pressing the car's pre-set buttons of my beloved stations, I have an ongoing personal relationship with my radio. Music from the 80s, NPR, the spa channel, talk radio like Insight are stations that I've chosen. I don't have to share the Entertainment Weekly channel or the Jenny McCarthy Show with anyone while I'm driving by myself. I listen to these programs so regularly that I feel I know the broadcasters more intimately than some acquaintances. I've stopped and listened to the Diane Rehm Show so many times and learned things I didn't even realize existed. I have a greater understanding of American culture when I hear about it from so many perspectives from the various stations. I'm getting reacquainted with songs I haven't heard in twenty years and being exposed to new music even before it's heard on FM radio.

XM radio has saved me on those days when I've felt alone, restless or even slightly bored with my routine. On any given driving trip, I can cry, laugh and sing thanks to my radio. More importantly, listening to radio has allowed my imagination to soar and my thought processes to broaden. Because there is nothing to look at or watch when listening to the radio, my mind has the freedom to travel on a path of its' own, one far away from the world of cancer and worry I've been living for the past two years. Every pause or nuance in the broadcaster's voice allows my mind to anticipate, ruminate or imagine. I walk away from my radio thinking more deeply about what I just heard. Many times, I'm anxious to tell my friends about what I listened to that day. It's no wonder that I often reference XM when I'm speaking to others about various topics. Even though it's not true, I tell my husband that I feel like I'm getting smarter thanks to my subscription.

In terms of my recovery, this radio couldn't have come at a better time. Upon hearing an interview with an author of a book on PTSD, I ran out and got the book to read. I'm somehow able to connect with the issues and narratives I hear about on a more empathetic level because of where I've been. I've Googled the names of writers, actors, musicians, bloggers, academics, critics and doctors whom I've heard speak on the radio to better understand their insights and help inform my own. When I hear the struggles those on the radio have gone through I'm able to put my own in a healthier context. Strangely, listening to the stories of others takes me both out my head but deeper into my thoughts. And that's a comfortable and humbling place for me to be.

March 21, 2015

32 THE KINDNESS OF STRANGERS

A few weeks ago I had an idea about writing a reflection on being stared at by strangers. It's something that I've been experiencing for almost two years and it had been on my mind. When I'm walking with my cane, I have a distinct gait that people not only notice but stare at. And without my cane, I walk with such a noticeable limp that if you watch me closely it looks like I could lose my balance at any given moment. Maybe this is why people are watching me so closely. They're waiting to see if I need help.

At some point, however, I abandoned the idea of writing about being stared at. Maybe it's because I've resigned myself to the fact that although the staring makes me uncomfortable there's nothing I can do about it. I'm not the only cane-toting, limping person out there in the world attracting the stares of others. People with all sorts of disabilities, restrictions, and afflictions are being stared at, too.

So this past week I decided to try something different. I tried reframing the way I look at the gawking strangers in my midst. And the biggest thing I did was the opposite of what I normally do when I'm walking past someone and feel his or her eyes watching me. Instead of relying on my default posture of looking downward and away from the stranger's eyes, I decided to make eye contact with the person. And while I certainly didn't stare at him or her, I didn't turn away either. The first few times I tried this I noticed the return of that recurring feeling I get of wanting to minimize myself. As tempting as it was to look away, I forced myself not to. So I practiced (and faked) feeling confident even if I wasn't. I tried to share pleasantries such as smiles and "good mornings" to passersby like I used to do all the time before my diagnosis and surgery. I stopped the chatter going on inside my head by silencing the self-pity and anger. I chose to step outside of myself and focus on the stranger standing in front of me.

And what I noticed is that people are kind. Many people are empathetic. Some people want to help. And so many of them are patient. I've watched as many strangers hold doors open for me even when there's a handicap button to press. I've appreciated people letting me in front of them in long line-ups. So many people have bent down to pick up my fallen cane that I've lost count. People smile back at me when I smile at them. When I walk away from these encounters what I feel most is my heart filling with gratitude.

So strangers stare at me. But when I allow it, their kindness embraces me. I feel like I've taken another baby step on the path towards self-acceptance. I hope.

April 11, 2015

33 THIS IS ME

Lately, it feels as if I've been losing touch with my identity as a person-in-recovery. I should qualify that and say my self-identity. The stronger I get and the better I feel, I'm sensing a renewal of sorts. Like a shedding of skin or a fresher coat of polish, I'm not sure, but slowly a new me is surfacing.

No amazing leaps in recovery have taken place allowing me to reach this point. I'm still walking with a cane. My limp is as pronounced as ever. Walking long distances remains both an elusive dream and a distant memory. Pain grips me on a consistently inconsistent basis. I'm not feeling any growth in my progression towards one day walking without an aid. Physically speaking,

I'm not any different than I was a month ago.

So I think about what has changed. And the only thing I come up with is an acceptance of where I am. For almost two years now I've forced myself to recite the Joseph Campbell quote that's been sitting to the left of my laptop. *We must let go of the life we have planned, so as to accept the one that is waiting for us.* Have I finally been able to do so, I wonder? As I take walks in my neighborhood gripping onto my walking poles with all my might, I say to myself, *this is me* instead of *I'm so tired of walking like this.* When I get the urge to join my kids outside and play on their scooters or tumble on the trampoline with them and I know I can't, I just sit out there and watch them. And I've been enjoying it more than I thought. When those pangs of grief start to surface, I take deep breaths and let them be.

This is me. These three powerful words have recently started coming to me whenever I sense resistance, sorrow, anger, or loss rising from within. I'm tired of fighting it. I know I can't reverse what's happened. I'm done with asking why me. I hope.

May 4, 2015

34 SECOND ANNIVERSARY APPROACHING

The twentieth of June is just around the corner. While I haven't been reliving those days leading up to my surgery in my mind as much as I did this time last year, I'm looking back at the last two years from a different perspective.

Striding in front of the mirror these days, I notice my posture is stronger and slightly straighter and I immediately remember my leaning and stooped stance post-surgery. I walk by my couch and get a vision of when my battered body lay on it for hours a day throughout that summer of 2013. I remember my husband's help putting on my socks and getting me in and out of the car in those early days. And

I still can recall the feeling of having my life scattered right in front of me and not knowing which piece to pick up first. Looking backwards, I see the growth, emotional and physical, that has taken place. And I am ever grateful. Without gratitude, I don't know where I'd be.

Yet here I am writing this entry today because I'm feeling down. It's like a reminder that despite the distances I've come, sadness will sometimes plague me. I've not been cured from melancholy. Maybe the gloom is necessary to my experiencing the joy? I need to embrace this heaviness, I remind myself. It might be trying to tell me something, and it probably is.

Yesterday I was reading a Young Adult novel and one of the young characters said something to another character who was going through a tough time that was so wise and true that it caught me off guard. He said something to the effect that *"this won't last forever"* and that *"you'll be in the dark for as long as it takes and then you'll come out*". I wish someone would've said these words to me two years ago. Living through that darkness, I remember, I couldn't see a way out. What I like most about this quote is the phrase "as long as it takes" because it honors the process: the embracing, the surrendering, and the moment of being exactly where you are.

June 16, 2015

35 MY FAMILY

This final piece is for Carlo, Annabel, and Karina.

How far I've come since March of 2013 is thanks to the three of you. I know that I wouldn't be hobbling around, preparing to return to work, travelling, laughing again, writing and enjoying life if I didn't have my family with me these past two years. You've been more than witnesses to my recovery. You've all played a major role in it.

Annabel, you were ten years old when I came home from the hospital in June 2013 and you had to watch your immobilized mother become so dependent on others. But you did far more than watch because you helped me so much in those early weeks. I remember the many times you'd be the "leg lifter" when I'd be trying to lie down on the couch or bed and couldn't lift my own leg. You were gentle and strong at the same time, taking on the job willingly and lovingly. I could see in your eyes how much you cared for me and felt badly for me. Over the past two years, you've grown into a mature and responsible person and I tend to think that my surgery and recovery somehow accelerated that process for you. I also want to thank you for doing things I know you didn't necessarily feel up to doing but you did them anyways because I couldn't. Running into the library for me, climbing loads of stairs to get me things, washing the floors (ugh!) and cutting trips to the mall short because my leg started to hurt. I remember these and apologize for the ways my illness has disrupted your and Karina's young lives.

Karina, you too have helped me in more ways than you know. Many times, you became my arms and legs: reaching, lifting, carrying, and grabbing. But more than anything else, my little one, you held me. You allowed me to cuddle up to you while lying on the couch reading the book *Gangsta Granny* together in those early weeks following my surgery. That despite the crutch or cane in my one hand, you always want to hold my other one when we're out walking. Your touch has been healing. It has made me feel loved. I remember us playing "chiropractor and patient" together and you were the doctor lifting my leg for counts of six. I could see how much you enjoyed the charge of helping me. Maybe my illness has helped bring out this compassionate side of you. Your patience, and Annabel's, is also what I'm grateful for. It couldn't have been easy missing out on fun things because your mom couldn't do them. I imagine that there are better ways of walking through Times Square in New York City than holding onto the side of your mother's wheelchair. But, you and your sister never complained. I was allowed to heal as well as

I have because of the two of you and your father.

Carlo, your world upended as quickly as mine did following my diagnosis. Together, we were thrust into a world neither of us ever would've imagined we'd be in. All of a sudden, you had me to worry about while holding the fort down for our young girls, never letting on to them how scared we were. Overnight, you became "Gina's Rock" and "Super-dad" at the same time. Your life was put on hold to take care of mine. And how you took it on . . . coming to all of my medical appointments, pushing my wheelchair for miles on end, cooking my meals, taking on my chores, helping me bathe, holding me at night while I cried, and taking care of our children's needs. And, you never once complained. I'll always remember you helping me get in and out of the therapy pool in those early months, even when the water was colder than you liked. How you had to put up with me on the days my pain stopped me (and us) in our tracks. Your positive spirit never wavered especially when mine used to. I miss the things we used to do together like taking long walks, cross country skiing, bike riding and in line skating. You lost your active partner and for this, I'm sorry. Thank you for everything you do for me. I love you.

I have many hopes moving forward. One is that my recovery is showing us all what a little strength and a lot of perseverance can do. I hope that the memories you three have of me while in the hospital and post-surgery will fade a bit but that the memories of you watching me slowly get better, one day at a time, won't disappear. There have been some life lessons for all of us in this journey. Life is precious, all we have is this moment, love is everything.

As ready as I now feel to move forward, I never want to forget the process (the good, the bad and the ugly) of getting to where I am today. A new me has emerged. A disabled, humbled, slightly wiser but definitely stronger me.

June 27, 2015

36 EPILOGUE

I'm a hypocrite. At least, it felt like I was this past summer. While vacationing in Hawaii, leg pain so severe and constant plagued me daily. Pinching, burning, gripping pain immobilized me. And that pain disconnected me from any reason, hope or acceptance that I've talked about throughout this book. Lying by the pool I'd imagine the relief I'd feel if this leg were severed from the rest of my body and replaced with a full prosthetic leg. An artificial leg that would be free of the pain-producing muscles and nerves that I have in my leg. I even made a mental note to ask my surgeon at my next visit about the possibility of a full leg replacement that I hoped would free me from the agony I was in. To hell with acceptance and my newly adopted "this is me" attitude. I wanted out.

That is, until I met a young woman one evening walking on a Honolulu sidewalk with a full prosthetic leg intact. I'd never met anyone in my travels nor at home with a full leg prostheses so I knew I had to speak with her. I had questions to ask her. I needed a close up look at what my future leg might look like and do. So in my wheelchair, I approached this young woman and introduced myself. Standing above me, she looked down at me and briefly shared her story.

Battling disease for the last eleven years, it was only this past January when doctors told her the leg had to come off. Six months with her new right leg and there she was walking in Hawaii. She explained to me the mechanics of the leg, the next steps required in her full transition to the leg and her life at home living with it. With pride, she told me how two days after she came home from the hospital following her amputation, she was driving a car using her left foot. I fired off as many questions I could think of and she, in turn, asked me about my story. In the end, we wished each other the best of luck and went our separate ways.

And like a ton of bricks, it hit me. I didn't want an artificial leg. I wanted my own. This one. Because beneath this young woman's positive spirit and enthusiasm, I sensed she was living with pain of her own. I understood that the grass wasn't any greener underneath her prosthetic limb than beneath my limping and aching one.

Later that night when we got back to our hotel, I was looking at my leg in the mirror while putting on my nightgown, and for the first time ever, I reached down and gave my left thigh a little rub and a tender pat. A huge wave of gratitude and love for everything this poor leg has to go through washed over me.

I know what I have to do. I have to mourn the "old" Gina and the ways she used to live. I have to make room for the "new" Gina, dogged by pain, who's been waiting patiently for me to fully accept her. I understand now that overcoming physical challenges takes time, lots of time. I've heard said that when the spirit is strong, the body will follow.

I have to keep my spirit strong.

August 23, 2015

ABOUT THE AUTHOR

Gina Luongo is the author of two published novels and a peer-reviewed paper and is currently working on a collection of short stories. She lives with her husband and two daughters in Toronto.